D1781875

```
362.1                    56490
Pau
Paullin, Ellen
Ted's stroke
```

Robinson Township Library
Robinson, Illinois 62454

Ted's Stroke

Ted's Stroke

The Caregiver's Story

by Ellen Paullin

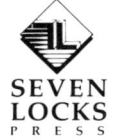

SEVEN LOCKS PRESS

Cabin John, Md./Washington, D.C.

Copyright © 1988 by Ellen Paullin

Library of Congress Cataloging-in-Publication Data
Paullin, Ellen, 1915—
   Ted's stroke: the caregiver's story/Ellen Paullin
     p. cm.
   Bibliography: p.
   Includes index.
   ISBN 0-932020-54-2 (alk. paper): $14.95
   1. Paullin, Theodore—Health.   2. Paullin, Ellen, 1915- .
   3. Cerebrovascular disease—Patients—United States—
      Biography.
   4. Cerebrovascular disease—Patients—Rehabilitation.
      I. Title.
RC388.5.P38P38   1988
362.1'9681'00924—dc19
[B]   88-1972
                                                                                                 CIP

Design and composition by Chuck Myers
American Labor Education Center

Printing and binding by Maple Vail Press

This book has been set in 11-pt. Century Oldstyle type and printed on acid-free paper.

Manufactured in the United States of America.

First printing, April 1988

SEVEN LOCKS PRESS
Publishers
P.O. Box 27
Cabin John, Md 20818
(301) 320-2130

Distributed to the trade by National Book Network,
Lanham, MD.

*To my best friend,
Ted Paullin,
and to the Writers Group,
who persuaded me
to tell our story*

Credits: The first five chapters of this book appeared, with some modifications, in *Northeast,* the magazine of the *Hartford Courant,* Hartford, Conn., October 13, 1985, under the title "The Story of a Stroke."

The lines from Emily Dickinson that appear throughout this book are from *The Complete Poems of Emily Dickinson,* edited by Thomas H. Johnson. Copyright 1914, 1929, 1935, 1942 by Martha Dickinson Bianchi. Copyright © renewed 1957, 1963 by Mary L. Hampson. By permission of Little, Brown and Co. Reprinted by permission of the publishers and trustees of Amherst College from *The Poems of Emily Dickinson,* edited by Thomas H. Johnson, Cambridge, Mass.: The Belknap Press of Harvard University Press, Copyright 1951, © 1955, 1979, 1983 by the President and Fellows of Harvard College.

The lines from "The First Snowfall" on pages 42-43 are from *The Poetical Works of James Russell Lowell,* vol. 4 (Cambridge, Mass.: Houghton Mifflin & Co., Riverside Press, 1904), p. 167.

The lines from "On His Blindness" by John Milton on page 43 are from *The Standard Book of British and American Verse,* selected by Nella Braddy (Garden City, N.Y.: Garden City Publishing Co., 1932), p. 137.

The quotation on page 53 is from *Deadeye Dick* by Kurt Vonnegut (New York, N.Y.: Dell Publishing Co., 1982), p. 208.

The lines from "The Deserted Village" by Oliver Goldsmith on page 115 appear in *Familiar Quotations,* ed. John Bartlett (Boston, Mass.: Little, Brown and Co., 1938), p. 250.

The lines from "Darius Green and His Flying Machine" by John Townsend Trowbridge on page 116 may be found in *The Book of Humorous Verse,* compiled by Carolyn Wells (Garden City, N.Y.: Garden City Publishing Co., 1936), p. 692.

Acknowledgments

For their invaluable suggestions and encouragement: Ruth Kurtz Alexander, Dr. Mary Elizabeth Fowler, Beth Hugh, Eric Johnson, Dr. Hugh Johnson, Tottie Johnson, Marcia Paullin, Dr. Susan Payne, Dr. Jane Satter, Lucy Townsend, Karen Paullin Will, Dr. Arthur Wolf.

The Writers Group: Beverly Berman, Brian Burland, Oliver Butterworth, Constance Carrier, Linda Case, Mary Hess, Christine Lyman Farquhar, Penn Ritter, Robert Satter, Ardis Whitman Rumsey.

Ellen Payne Paullin
Newington, Connecticut
January 1988

Contents

I.	**The Sirens Were for Him** *Events leading up to the stroke* *The emergency room*	3
II.	**A Short History: Ted and Ellen**	14
III.	**Life Revolves Around the ICU** *Companions in ICU* *Relations with doctors and nurses*	20
IV.	**New Horizons:** **The Skilled Nursing Facility** *Therapy* *Preparations for homecoming*	31
V.	**A New and Different Daily Life** *Home care* *Wheelchair living* *Cataract operation* *Reading patterns* *Talking Books*	37
VI.	**The Nitty-Gritty**	44
VII.	**"The Story of a Stroke"**	56
VIII.	**The Phenomenon of Support Groups** *The Stroke Club* *The Voluntary Stroke Rehabilitation Program*	66

IX.	**Adult Day Care**	80
	Activities	
	A visit to another day care center	
X.	**Problems: Financial and Otherwise**	91
	Financial problems for the disabled and/or elderly	
	Caring for the caregiver	
XI.	**Journeying in '86**	100
	Panama Canal cruise	
	Michigan—Breadloaf—Wisconsin	
XII.	**January '87 Setback**	108
XIII.	**Coping**	122

Afterwords

A Physician's Retrospective
Dr. Arthur D. Wolf — 133

Stroke! *Dr. Alan S. Greenglass* — 155

Appendix

Bibliography — 165

Suggested Readings
On Stroke/Cerebrovascular Disease — 165
On Zone Therapy — 167
Personal Narratives — 167
Publications — 168

Additional Information
Day Care — 168
Travel Information — 169

Index — 171

Ted's Stroke
The Caregiver's Story

The Paullin Family
1984

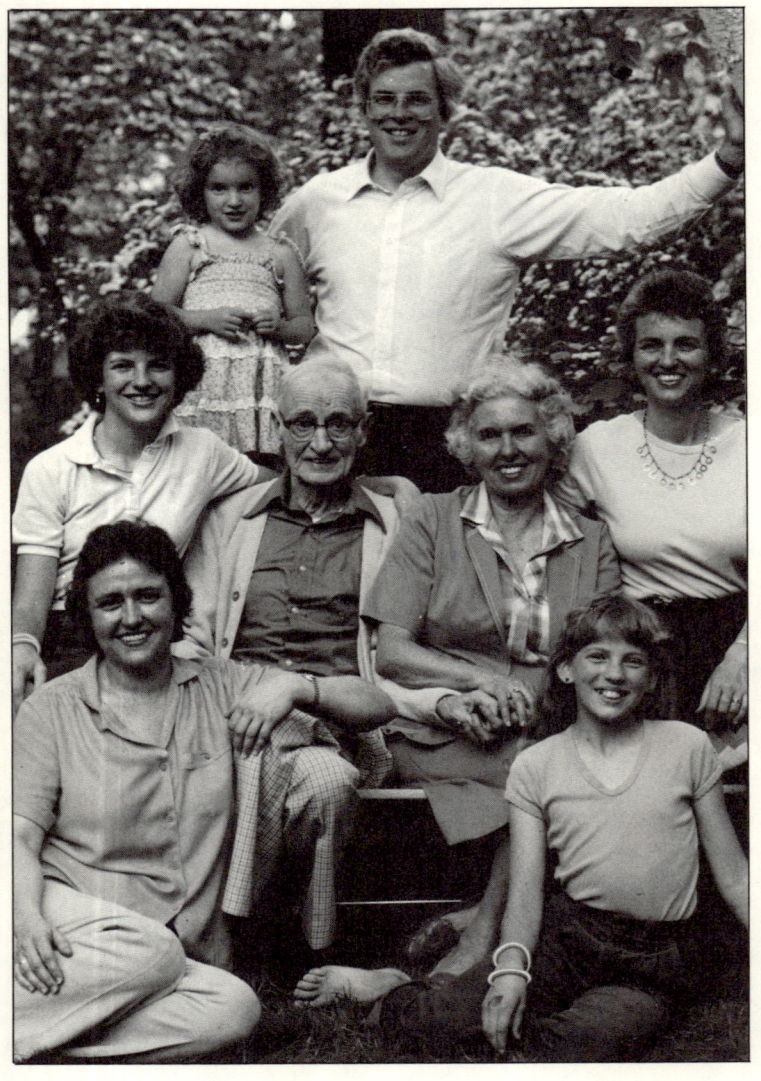

Colleen Will   Philip Will
Kayden Will   Ted and Ellen Paullin   Karen Paullin Will
Marcia Paullin   Bryn Will

CHAPTER I

The Sirens Were for Him

Elysium is as far as to
The very nearest Room
If in that Room a Friend await
Felicity or Doom—

What fortitude the Soul contains,
That it can so endure
The accent of a coming Foot—
The opening of a Door—

—Emily Dickinson

"Wow! A disc camera. Excellent! Just what I wanted. Thank you, Grandpa, thank you."

Nine-year-old Bryn, the birthday girl, reached over and hugged Ted, her long blonde hair falling across his face and hiding his pleased smile. All of us clapped as she said, "Now my first picture is going to be of all of you guys. Get together over on the couch, there. C'mon, Coleen, get on Grandpa's lap. Grandma, you sit on the other side of Grandpa."

I moved as directed, delighted to be following directions since I usually was on the other end of the process, bossing people into positions for photographs, listening to their protests, enduring their groans. Hearing Bryn call out instructions to her sisters, her parents, and to us was a new experience, and we all sat erect and expectant—her mother (our daughter Karen); Karen's husband, Phil; eleven-year-old Kayden; and two-year-old

Colleen—crowding close together and putting on our smiling picture faces. As Bryn found the small button and pressed it, the flash went off.

"Wow, everything is automatic. Excellent." (Her fad word of the year again.) "Now I want just Grandpa and Colleen. They look good together." We all moved aside as she gave orders about how Grandpa was to put his arms around his squirming grandchild. Just as she was ready to take the picture, Ted leaned over and kissed Colleen on top of her curls.

"Wow, that's neat," exclaimed Bryn. Later, she took quiet pride in telling everyone in the family, "I did it with my new camera. I took the last picture before he..."

Gently placing Colleen beside him on the couch, Ted turned to me. "If I leave now, I can get home in time to see the Packers play." I nodded perfunctorily, remembering that from early morning he had been reminding me of the football game at nine that night. We had come in two cars, from different meetings; if he left now, I would be able to stay to hear Kayden play her recital piece. "Fine," I said. "See you in a little while."

Before he left, Ted gave Bryn a big hug. " 'Bye, Brynnie. I'm looking forward to all those pictures you're going to take."

"So am I, Grandpa, so am I," she said enthusiastically, returning his hug.

About forty-five minutes later, as I was getting ready to leave, Colleen came up, carrying her jacket, and grabbed me around the knees. "I going to your house, too."

For a moment I saw in my mind the only beautiful, blank day on my September calendar. I had counted on tomorrow, a whole unscheduled block of time, to read,

The Sirens Were for Him

write, walk—a day without interruptions. Colleen's being there would change all that. But the beauty of the empty calendar square suddenly faded as I remembered my friend saying just that afternoon, "How lucky you are to be near your children." And another had said with envy, "How I wish I could watch my grandchild grow up!"

I swooped Colleen up in my arms, ran to the car, and started to drive the five familiar miles from Hartford to our suburb.

A soft, gentle rain had begun, enough to cover the streets with a thin film of wetness that reflected every light along the way. As I drove up the hill toward our driveway, I was startled to see that Ted's car wasn't there. The blank space where it should have been almost shouted at me. Hurrying into the house, Colleen behind me, I went from room to room, from basement to attic, calling. Perhaps he had gone to Buddy's, his colleague in the history department who shared his enthusiasm for the football team from Green Bay, Wis., where Ted had grown up. A call produced "No, haven't heard a word from him since our card game."

I remembered the shimmering lights on the wet streets; Ted must have had an accident. Because of a cataract in one eye, he didn't have binocular vision and disliked driving at night. I began calling the police, first in our town, then in the city. No—no recently reported accidents. Then I called the emergency rooms at the two nearest hospitals. No—no new admissions. What *could* have happened?

I called Karen to report to her, hoping desperately that Ted had had some delay and had gotten in touch with her. She had heard nothing, but her voice began to reflect the anxiety in mine. "I'll ask Phil to get in our car and drive along the way Dad would have gone." I agreed that that would be a good idea although I had just driven that way myself.

Standing at our front door, wondering what to do next, I heard ambulance sirens nearby. I knew they could have nothing to do with Ted, for he had left Karen's more than an hour ago. Suddenly Phil appeared at the back door.

"He's had a stroke," he said, in his calm, quiet way. "He's been taken to the hospital. We'll go there right now."

I called Karen and our close friend, Arthur Wolf, a physician on the hospital staff. Shocked by my message, both said they would meet us in the ER (emergency room) as soon as possible.

"Ted pulled his car off to the side of the road in that construction section up there opposite the Texaco station," Phil reported. "When I got there, the police were in charge and the ambulance was just leaving." He got Colleen's jacket and took her to his car. I followed in my car, impatient at stop signs, resenting traffic slowed by the rain.

The sirens—I shuddered—they *had* been for him. He had been only a mile from our house. Suddenly, I was overwhelmed as I realized I had driven right by his car on my way home, just a short half-hour before. Ted had been helpless, perhaps in pain, probably dying, and I, talking with Colleen and paying attention to the wet road in front of me, hadn't seen the familiar blue car off at the side of the street. How long had he been there? If I had stopped, would I have known what to do? Where would I have gone for help?

The ER seemed too quiet, too calm, too organized to

hold the traumatic news I expected to hear. Karen was sitting in a little corner room. Suddenly she and Phil and I were holding each other closely with Colleen crushed somewhere in the middle.

Arthur Wolf, our doctor friend, came to us immediately from a cubicle across the room and answered our urgent, unspoken question. "Yes, he is breathing. I've called in a neurologist who can help us find out where the damage is. Just now, though, Ted's heart is strong."

"How could he have a strong heart?" Karen asked. "He never believed in exercise."

"They used to ask him if he'd run the 440 in high school every time they did a physical on him—his heart was so slow," I added.

"Slow, but strong," said Arthur, reassuringly.

I decided to call Marcia, our younger daughter, even before we had any more news of Ted's condition. As we expected, she said she would leave immediately and drive from Philadelphia straight to the hospital.

Phil left for home with Colleen as Karen and I sat down to wait. She reminded me of the perfect weekend Ted had just had: his game of set-back on Friday (an old card game, sometimes known as "schmeer" or "high, low, jack, and the game," which he had played monthly for thirty-six years), a retreat in the country with Quaker friends on Sunday, a birthday celebration with his family on Monday. "If it's got to be an ending, it's a fitting one," she said, philosophically.

I had talked with her earlier that evening, expressing a longing for some "alone time" in this household with two retirees. In a moment, she added to her remark about "a fitting ending." "Now you may have 'alone time' with a vengeance."

We anxiously watched the closed cubicle where Ted lay. Finally, it opened and we were given a signal to come. The unconscious, pale figure on the upraised bed had tubes in his nose and arms; a respirator was puffing away at his side. Karen began talking to him, assuring him of our presence and our concern. I pulled off the sheets at the end of the bed and began rubbing his feet.

"This is the spot that corresponds to your heart, Ted. You're going to be all right."

"Hey, his finger moved," exclaimed Karen.

"That's good," said one of the nurses. "We're going to do a brain scan now to see where the hemorrhage was. We'll take him upstairs for that. You can wait in the lounge on the seventh floor."

After what seemed to us a long, long time, Arthur brought us the news that the scan revealed a hemorrhage in the cerebellum. After consulting with the neurologist, he had called in a neurosurgeon, who advised surgery as soon as possible.

I signed the necessary papers, and Karen and I settled ourselves in the lounge near the ICU (intensive care unit) for neurosurgical patients. In those dark, quiet hours, we were each compiling our own lists of "Why didn't I . . ."

Among all the major regrets, one little one kept popping into my mind, and I realized it had been nagging me ever since we got to the hospital. For weeks the latch on the door to our screen-house in the backyard had been broken. Finally, just yesterday, Ted had fixed it by finding a square wooden drawer knob and cleverly attaching it to the door. I had not expressed one word of appreciation or admiration for the job he had done. I knew it had meant a lot to him to spend his time figuring out that kind of problem, so different from the time he usually spent reading the latest best-sellers or his French novels, or doing his double-crostics. And I had ignored his achievement. I suddenly remembered Emily Dickinson's

> *Remorse is cureless-the Disease*
> *Not even God-can heal*

I had always thought that poem might haunt me some day when I would remember large omissions as well as small ones.

The neurosurgeon appeared about two in the morning, tired but smiling.

"He came through the operation very well. He's had an intracerebellar hemorrhage; he will probably have deficits in coordination but his cognitive functions are not affected," he explained tersely. As I thanked him, I had a vision of myself pushing a wheelchair down a long, narrow path for the rest of our lives, and I smiled in relief as I knew how gladly I would settle for that if only Ted's mind would be as keen as it had always been.

At Karen's, where I spent the remaining part of the night, I fell into bed exhausted, but before sleeping I had a sudden image of the tickets to New Zealand and Australia that were lying on Ted's desk: stopovers in Perth, Alice Springs, Melbourne, and Sydney; a jeep trip to the Outback to see aboriginal cave drawings; a visit to the Great Barrier Reef. Now I'd have to tell Edith, our travel agent, that all the hours she had spent arranging schedules, tours, hotels, and planes had been for nothing.

Shortly after six in the morning, Marcia woke me, bounding up the stairs and shouting, "He squeezed my hand, he opened his eyes, he saw me."

There are not many courses in the curriculum called "Coping with Catastrophe." Surely we had had no preparation, but we knew we had to begin our "one-day-at-a-time" existence. Marcia took a week off from her teaching; we called a friend in Pennsylvania to come stay with Karen's children. We began our daily vigils at the hospital.

I knew that I was missing a lot of phone calls at home but hadn't yet made use of the efficient, mechanical solution to that problem. Phil and Karen installed a phone-answering machine for me, and I began to look forward to listening to messages from the hosts of friends and relatives who called to express their care and concern. I could also leave information about Ted's condition, which is what they wanted. I resolved never again to rationalize *not* expressing concern ("they are probably tired of too many calls," "she is probably resting," "one more card won't mean anything") for the calls, the cards and letters, the flowers all offered me tangible support at the end of the day. As I reported each one to Ted, his eyes filled with tears.

Many times that week we relied upon the healing power of laughter, so well described in Norman Cousins's book, *The Anatomy of an Illness*. It came in small but significant doses.

In retrospect, we could even laugh at what we called "the third-day syndrome": Karen was arrested for making a left turn where it was prohibited, Marcia was fined for forgetting to feed the hospital parking meter, and I was stopped by a policewoman for going the wrong way on a one-way street.

"But my husband is in intensive care—he had a stroke," I explained, frantically.

"Lady, if you're that distraught, you shouldn't be driving."

The Sirens Were for Him

We were puzzled one day when Ted began to move one hand back and forth to his mouth. One of the first questions we had been asked in the ER was "Does he smoke?" He was seventy-two and he had stopped twelve years earlier, but for thirty-four years, he had smoked rather heavily. Now he seemed to be making signs that he wanted a cigarette. The doctor explained that this was very natural, for when brain functions return, they do so chronologically. Ted was probably at about the period when he was used to smoking when he felt frustrated. It occurred to us, then, that Karen must look very much the way I looked forty years ago when he was smoking a lot.* He probably thought *she* was his wife and wondered what in the world this old gray-haired woman was doing, hanging around his room all the time!

I was hanging around the room as often as I could, trying to think of ways to communicate with Ted. Since he was unable to swallow, feeding tubes ran through his nose into his stomach, which must have been very uncomfortable. At one count, an intern told us, he had pulled the tubes out thirteen times. To discourage this, they had bound his hands with mitts of gauze and tied his wrists to the bed.

"The last time, even when his hands were tied, he scooted down in the bed and pulled the damn tubes out

---

*According to research by Dr. Robert D. Abbott, biostatistician at the National Heart, Lung and Blood Institute in Bethesda, Md., cigarette smokers are far more likely than nonsmokers to have strokes, but they can reduce their risk significantly by giving up the habit. Of the 500,000 people who have strokes each year, 156,000 die. This represents a 30 percent decrease in the death rate over the last twenty years, probably due in part to an increasing number of people who have given up smoking.

with his knees," one exasperated resident complained.

"Bully for Ted," I thought. "He's okay." That was unfair, I know, for it was a horrible job to reinsert the tubes, but I also understood the patient who wanted them out.

I remember wondering at the time whether Ted's actions could have been the result of the painfulness of the tubes, or had he recalled our conversations about "pulling the tubes" or "unplugging the life-support systems" when hope was gone. Either motivation seemed reasonable to me—not evidence of "irrational behavior," as the doctor described it later.

The bulky gauze mitts further hindered the only communication we had established: "If you hear me, squeeze my hand." The squeezes had been compared daily for intensity, duration, and warmth, and now they were denied us.

I decided to buy magnetic alphabet letters on a board to see if Ted could spell out words. In a store called Creative Playtime, the woman in front of me was buying a toy to put her child to sleep.

"It will not always be your problem," I assured her. "I'm buying a toy to keep an elderly gentleman awake."

A great breakthrough in understanding came about the third week after Ted entered the hospital. In the summer, he had been named to the board of directors of the Alexander Meiklejohn Experimental College Foundation. I brought a letter he had received from one of the officers to read to him, and I noticed the new letterhead listing the board members, all of whom had been in the Experimental College at the University of Wisconsin with him. I began to read the names aloud. On the spur of the moment, about halfway down the list, I decided to test his alertness. I threw in a made-up name, without skipping a beat: "Richard Limbocker."

Ted slowly shook his head, "No, no." I shrieked with joy. If you exist anywhere on this planet, Richard Limbocker, I love you greatly.

CHAPTER II

A Short History: Ted and Ellen

*I measure every Grief I meet
With narrow, probing, Eyes—
I wonder if It weighs like Mine—
Or has an Easier size.*

—Emily Dickinson

As I left Ted's room that day, I thought of Alexander Meiklejohn, the renowned educator who had founded that Experimental College, which had meant so much to Ted. When I got home I looked up a definition I had seen in one of his books:

> Intelligence... is readiness for any human situation; it is the power, wherever one goes, of being able to see, in any set of circumstances, the best response which a human being can make to those circumstances.*

If only we could have that kind of power in the days ahead of us!

Ted was the only son of a Baptist minister who was serving a church in Denver, Colo., when Ted was born in 1910. In World War I, the minister deserted his wife and child, and Ted's mother became one of the pioneers in what we now call "single parenthood." Having taught

---

*Alexander Meiklejohn, *The Experimental College*, ed. and abr. by John Walker Powell (Cabin John, Md.: Seven Locks Press, 1981), p.5.

Ted and Ellen

for a few years after graduating from eighth grade, she returned to her home and continued teaching in elementary schools in Green Bay, Wis., for the next twenty-five years.

When Ted went to the University of Wisconsin at Madison in the fall of 1927, she gave him half her salary each month (*half* of $150.00) so he could study full time without having to get a job. He worked summers at a soda fountain in a Door County summer resort while his mother was employed there as a housekeeper.

As a freshman on a very limited budget, he discovered that if he joined ROTC (Reserve Officers' Training Corps) the Army would issue him a uniform; this he could wear three days a week and thus get by with only one other suit. He didn't think much about what ROTC was for until the day the class was maneuvering in a big open field near the university.

"Shoot 'em in the legs, boys," the army sergeant ordered. "It takes two to carry 'em off the field."

Suddenly the nature of what he was being trained for dawned on him. From that day on he has embraced pacifism, and its values have been the core of his personal beliefs.

I'm sure he has been sustained by his unusual educational experience during his freshman and sophomore years at the University of Wisconsin's Experimental College (1927-32), which was housed in one of the campus dormitories. Ted was one of a hundred students who participated in the first class of this unique curriculum, studying fifth-century Athens in their first year and nineteenth-century America in their second. There were no formal classes and no grades, but students met weekly with individual advisers (among them, historian Carl Russell Fish, political scientist John Gaus, writer

Francis Steegmuller, and classicist Walter Agard) to discuss required papers, and they had many opportunities to talk about their assignments with fellow students in seminars. Outstanding speakers—Bertrand Russell, Frank Lloyd Wright, Irish poet AE (George William Russell), and economist Walton Hamilton, among them—also visited the college. Encouraging his students to express every point of view, Alexander Meiklejohn offered an environment in which they were exposed to many.

For his junior and senior years and his M.A. and Ph.D. degrees, Ted attended the university proper, majoring in history. Then, after teaching one year at Park College in Parkville, Mo., he came to the University of Kansas at Lawrence, where I met him and where we were married. Ted registered as a conscientious objector in October 1940, a fact that became well known on campus and resulted in his having to leave his job in 1942.

The Pacifist Research Bureau, related to the American Friends Service Committee (Quakers) in Philadelphia, was being formed by Friends and others to research and publish programs for the peaceful world they hoped would follow the war. Ted was hired to write for the PRB,* so in 1942 we moved to Swarthmore, Pa., with five-week-old Karen. We later became members of the Friends Meeting there, discovering that we felt we had really been Quakers for a long time without an opportunity for formal affiliation.

I began teaching in the Friends School in nearby Media because we assumed Ted would be assigned to a camp for

---

*His publications include *An Introduction to Non-Violence*; *Comparative Peace Plans*; *Coercion of States: in Federal Unions*; *Coercion of States: in International Organizations* (co-author).

conscientious objectors when he was drafted and we would be responsible for his monthly expenses there. But the day before he was to go to C.O. camp he was notified that he should have a new physical exam. Because of deafness in one ear, he was classified "4-F" (physical disability for military service). We had already had his farewell party, complete with gifts of soap, sewing kits, and paperbacks. The warm support of the friends who had been at that party sustained us and surrounded us with a reassuring climate during the remaining years of the war.

After the war we moved from the security of that Quaker community to Connecticut, not knowing how our ideas would be accepted in "the land of steady habits." The respect and esteem of his colleagues at Central Connecticut State University, where Ted was professor of history from 1947 to 1978, have been a testament to his integrity and to their understanding. And in those years, Ted's dedication to peace motivated him to serve on many regional and national Quaker committees, and to spend two years in Paris as director of Quaker International Seminars in Europe.

I am pretty sure the direction Ted's life took was not one that could have been foreseen by that barking sergeant on the windy field by Lake Mendota years ago, but for Ted, it was the best response he could make to the situations in which he found himself, and I counted on that power serving him well in this new, unexpected, and possibly devastating experience with a stroke.

As for me, I would be facing our problems from a very different background. My childhood was more gregarious than Ted's (gregarious: "habitually living or moving in flocks or herds"). First of seven children, I was born in Amherst, Mass., in 1915. My father and mother had moved there from Oklahoma so Dad could take his first job as a member of the faculty at Massachusetts Agricultural College (now University of Massachusetts). Years later, in an American literature class, I discovered Emily Dickinson and realized that my "formative years" had been spent just around the corner from the house in which she had lived most of her life.

After five years in Amherst, our family moved to Manhattan, Kans., where I lived until I graduated from Kansas State University in 1936. In college I was active in the student YWCA, and the leaders in its summer conferences at Estes Park, Colo., inspired the values I have held ever since. In fact, only a few years after Ted was marching around the field in his ROTC uniform, I was picketing the ROTC office on our campus to protest the fact that ROTC training was compulsory.

Immediately after graduation, I became executive secretary of the student YWCA at the University of Kansas at Lawrence. There I met the new history instructor at a YWCA faculty-student tea. In our years at KU we were both active in the effort to integrate campus facilities (black students could not attend dances in the Student Union and were segregated in its dining rooms). We also formed a pacifist discussion group, which supported two of our students who were sent to camps for conscientious objectors after the United States entered the war. And we helped organize meetings for those who sought an economic system that would offer a better life for more people. One of those meetings culminated in a rally in the city park at which Norman Thomas, the Socialist candidate for president, spoke. It attracted a large and enthusiastic crowd in those days.

When our daughters were in school, I wrote several books for children, entered politics for a few years, and worked on many Quaker committees, including one that edited a hymnal and two songbooks for Friends. After the girls entered college, I worked for seventeen years in public relations at Hartford College for Women.

I retired in 1977, and after forty-three years of teaching, Ted taught his last class in 1978. How fortunate we were that his stroke occurred when we were living "scheduleless" days, when our home was paid for, when Ted's retirement pay was adequate for our living expenses, when our daughters were grown and able to care for themselves. Younger stroke victims would have much more difficult adjustments to make and incredibly greater worries in terms of careers and finances. And what if the caregiver were employed and had to squeeze the caregiving into the margins of daily life? Being able to be with Ted whenever he needed me would have been impossible if I'd been working.

I was aware of all this each day I returned to the hospital and met others who had friends or relatives in the ICU. Each patient—each family—faced a unique tragedy, but none of us was immune to pain. Indeed, it seemed as if it might have no end.

CHAPTER III

Life Revolves Around the ICU

*Pain—has an Element of Blank—
It cannot recollect
When it begun—or if there were
A time when it was not—*
 —*Emily Dickinson*

Visits to patients were limited to fifteen minutes each hour on the half-hour. Sometimes I thought I would never see any number but "6" on a clock face again.

The routine of our days became very closely associated with the lounge where we had spent such anxious hours that first night. The lounge became a second home but without any of the amenities of a home—or a civilized waiting room, for that matter. There were no magazines, no books, no lamps, no comfortable chairs, no freedom from incessant cigarette smoke (now changed), and no privacy. The community of the waiting place, however, created intense relationships. It became a curiously contained world, completely isolated from the normal comings and goings in the streets below, filled with a succession of heart-wrenching encounters.

The first night, as Karen and I awaited the results of Ted's surgery, a shadowy figure on the opposite side of the lounge pulled two chairs together and stretched out to try to sleep. She turned out to be the mother of a seventeen-year-old college freshman who had just had an operation for a brain tumor. The girl died four days after

Life Revolves Around the ICU

we had begun to share the long hours in the waiting room with her parents. Such closeness to a family, in such short time, we had never felt before.

Also on that first night, I talked with the wife of a young man who had fallen down the cellar stairs. "He was so worried about layoffs at the plant," she explained. "He would begin drinking when he came home. We got to arguing about the kids. . . . He stumbled and fell . . . real hard."

On the second day, we met a beautiful young woman whose thirty-three-year-old husband, father of their three boys, had started having severe headaches during the summer. After many tests, he was admitted to the hospital, where a brain tumor was discovered and removed; however, he never regained consciousness. She had lost her father when she was four and had always dreaded, more than anything else, the same loss befalling her own children who were now eight, six, and three. "And I don't even know how to show the boys how to tie a necktie," she sobbed.

One day a nineteen-year-old, who had been riding his bicycle home from work at midnight and had been struck by a hit-and-run driver, was brought to the ICU. His father, a French-Canadian ironworker, came with his wife and nine children, one of whom was the victim's identical twin, to spend the long hours waiting. After the boy's brain death, they discussed quietly in the lounge whether to donate his kidney to another patient.

A high school boy died soon after he was brought to the seventh floor. He had been beaten with a baseball bat by a gang of boys as he left a party. "It was a mistake," his older brother said softly. "They thought he was another guy."

In the second week I talked to the sister of a man

brought in with a crossbow arrow straight through his head. "He had no enemies; he was so well liked where he worked. His wife and three kids were asleep upstairs when it happened. Who could have done this.... How could it possibly...." The distraught sister's voice trailed off as she stared out the window. A year later, we were shocked to read that a jury had found the wife guilty of her husband's murder; she was sentenced by the judge to thirty-five years in prison.

Some of the patients whose families we met in the ICU recovered and were transferred to another part of the hospital, but Karen and I went to the funerals of the college freshman, the young father, and the nineteen-year-old cyclist. It was the natural expression of the bond we felt with the relatives whose lives we had touched so closely in those agonizing hours in the lounge. At times I felt guilty knowing I still had someone to visit when the clock hand got to "6"; at other times, thinking of the radically different future ahead for Ted and me, I wondered.

Karen and I described the effect of those first weeks in the hospital as the "yo-yo syndrome." One day the reports were despairing: "He's not quite up to what we thought he'd be at this time." The next day Ted would be giving us firm hand squeezes and listening to a baseball game on the radio. One morning we came in to find him sitting in a chair-with-wheels, which we were able to push down the hall; he waved to all the other patients. The next evening we arrived to find his bed surrounded by doctors. His breathing had stopped, and only the action of the nurse who quickly attached him to the respirator had saved him. One day he seemed to appreciate the cassettes we left on in his room—Rubinstein playing Brahms, and the Weavers' "Wasn't That a

Life Revolves Around the ICU

Time." The next day he was irritated and annoyed by music. It was hard to follow one doctor's advice: "You must paint this with a broad brush. Don't react minute by minute." But living one day at a time, one hour at a time, one minute at a time, was the only way we could survive. The daily seesawing was wearing, however, and I got small comfort from thinking "this, too, shall pass away" because it applied to the good times as well as to the bad.

During those unpredictable days, one of the most frustrating experiences was my difficulty in communicating with the doctors. Every bit of information about Ted's condition—his improvement or lack of it, his hopes for the future—had to be probed for and pried out of anyone attending him.

If I had had enough sleep the night before or had a moment of perspective, I could remind myself of the operation by the neurosurgeon at one in the morning, which had probably saved Ted's life. I could persuade myself that that tired surgeon was no doubt heading for the operating room to save other lives the very morning that I wanted him to talk with me; that it was not up to him to volunteer information if Ted was getting along satisfactorily; that the doctor's isolation was his only insulation against those of us who were begging for analysis and prognosis and, yes, emotional support. On rare days I realized my demands and expectations were unreasonable. On most days, I hadn't enough wisdom to be this considerate in my responses.

I was also unreasonable in my attitude toward the residents making rounds in their wrinkled blue coats, huddling together, whispering, smiling, nodding at each other, then turning blank faces to me as they passed, never offering information unless I interrupted them.

Nurses also offered little information: "Ask your doctor," they would say in a tone that could be interpreted equally as encouraging or ominous.

Ask your doctor? What doctor? I had called Arthur Wolf that first night because, as a very good friend, he had been with us through other health emergencies. (Ted's family doctor, who practiced in Newington, took over later when Ted returned there.) Arthur called in the neurologist and the neurosurgeon the night Ted entered the hospital. The latter called in the pulmonologist, who did a bronchoscopy; the pulmonologist called in an ear, nose, and throat man, who did a tracheotomy; he referred the swallowing problem to another surgeon, who eliminated the feeding tubes through the nose by doing a gastrostomy so Ted could be fed by a long tube inserted directly into his stomach. The problem of what to put into the tube was transferred to a nutrition-specialist, who referred the complications that arose after the tube feeding to a urologist.

When I complained about the impersonality, the unsatisfactory communication, and the accumulation of bills and paperwork, my friends said, "But surely you don't want that other option, one of those programs like an HMO. You don't get to *choose* your own doctor." Out of eight physicians, I had chosen only the first one, our friend. As soon as we became eligible, I filled out the application for Kaiser Permanente, the nearest health maintenance organization I could find. It was an insurance option possible for us at certain times of the year because of Ted's status as a retired state employee.

That decision was one of the wisest I made in all those months. I had had to spend from two to four mornings a week trying to sort out the bills and forms (each doctor had a different system), filling in blanks, calling the state

Life Revolves Around the ICU

retirement office to discover that they *didn't* cover what I thought they did, and calling Medicare and Social Security to discover that they *did* cover what I thought they didn't. The hours of paperwork—including the time spent making out checks and depositing income for the general running of the house, jobs Ted had always taken care of—were staggering.

But since the day our membership in Kaiser became effective, I have seen not one piece of paper, not one bill, not one form to fill in. The relief is compounded by the excellent patient-care procedures: "advice-nurses" answer the phone and solve minor problems, nurse practitioners see us for any non-emergency, and, most important to me, our doctor calls back to check up on any problem I have talked with the advice-nurse about! He has provided physical and speech therapists for Ted, and he sends him to specialists when he finds that necessary. The time I save is astronomical: no need to make special appointments and trips for X rays, blood tests, or eye tests—all are in the same compact headquarters; no more frantic trips to the library or post office to make copies of forms for the IRS, the insurance company, and always the one extra for my own files. I cannot speak too highly of this new approach to complete medical care.

Paperwork did not disappear entirely from my schedule, however, but from the beginning I chose a very different kind. When we left for the hospital the morning after Ted's stroke, I grabbed a pen and a bright red looseleaf notebook from Karen's desk. On the opening page was her first assignment for a French class she was auditing at a nearby college: to write a paper on what you did last summer, "deux pages, sautez une ligne." Well, she skipped many lines, for she never saw the notebook again. "This is history," I explained as we left the house, "and it must be recorded history." The notebook became my journal, absorbing faithfully all the outpourings it received each evening when I came home from the hospital.

One of the first entries was copied from the records in the West Hartford police department: it was the report of the policeman who found Ted in the car beside the road that rainy September night. Ted had pulled his car off the street in a section of West Hartford between Hartford and our suburb of Newington; I had not thought to call the West Hartford police the night of the stroke. This was the report:

Police Record #5903   Officer Dwyer

R (referred)   unknown person

Victim found sitting in front seat of vehicle having what appeared to be a stroke. Victim given oxygen; L&M Ambulance notified at 9:40. Arrived at 9:44. Departed at 9:48 for Hartford Hospital at request of victim. Hartford Hospital advised. When called victim is under emergency room treatment. Condition unknown. Victim's vehicle towed to Lou's Amoco station, 1056 New Britain Ave. Time of report 9:33. So. Street and Jansen Court, West Hartford. Sept. 20, 1982

I talked with Officer Dwyer by phone for I was puzzled by the phrase "at request of victim." We had assumed Ted had been unconscious when he was found.

"No," said the policeman, "he definitely wanted to be taken to Hartford Hospital."

"How do you determine whether there has been a stroke or a heart attack?" I asked.

"First thing we do is feel for a pulse. If there is one, it's

Life Revolves Around the ICU

a stroke. If there isn't any, it's a heart attack. As police, we can stop bleeding, give oxygen, or try to prevent shock, but usually we can give no other medical assistance. That's why I called the ambulance immediately."

I shuddered as I realized that, had I found Ted, I probably would have assumed a heart attack and would have tried, in my imperfect but desperate way, to give artificial respiration. Would those movements have dislodged a clot that could have been fatal? Or if I had run to the nearest house to use a phone, would they have let me in? Would I have known which ambulance to call? I'm sure I wouldn't have thought to call the police, who had such an efficient way of getting in touch with the ambulance and taking care of Ted's car.

Weeks later, Ted corroborated the fact that the policeman had stuck his head in the car window and asked, "Is anything wrong?" The last thing Ted remembers, from then until two months later, was his reply from the floor in the front seat of the car where he had fallen, "Do you think I'd be down here if everything was all right?"

The journal helps me remember that at the end of that first week I took our oldest granddaughter, Kayden, to see a local theater production of *On Borrowed Time,* in which the old grandfather manages to keep Death up in a tree so that he and his grandson can be together longer. Their final realization of how important death is in the world, and of what a dreadful place it would be without it, gave new perspective to those of us whose energies were concentrated on trying to prevent it from entering that room in the ICU just a few blocks away.

Bolstered by the play's message, Karen and I planned an appointment with the funeral director on the next weekend that Marcia came up from Philadelphia. All our questions about embalming, cremation, and types of service we might have were answered at a time when we knew we were going right back to the hospital to squeeze Ted's hand. We filled in forms for a service for both Ted and me, and the three of us left on that sunny morning grateful for the sympathetic, thoughtful person who had helped us face the unfaceable; we realized how much better we felt for having done it.

Crisis after crisis occurred in October: Ted's arms were "infiltrated" from the IVs; they were swollen, red, and feverish; and from wrist to shoulder they were blotched red and purple where blood had been taken. When asked about the rise in temperature noted on the chart, a resident said, "There seems to be a staph infection of some kind. But I guess you feel better about that than when they told you about his pneumonia a couple of days ago." No one had mentioned a word about pneumonia to us.

A few days later the doctor who was to do the gastrostomy reported that they had detected a heart murmur, the significance of which was not yet known, so they would have to postpone the operation. A bladder infection, which developed after the eventual gastrostomy, seemed par for the course.

Eventually the crises became more infrequent, and it began to look as if Ted, the longest remaining inhabitant in the ICU cubicles, could be moved to a room where he could be cared for by the regular nursing staff. Finally, at the end of the sixth week, he was moved to Room 729. We filled it with flowers and posters, and rejoiced at the expanded visiting hours.

He still needed to be suctioned for mucus in the tracheotomy tube whenever he coughed; speaking was very difficult. Gradually he gained enough strength to walk with an aide on each side; his balance was so impaired that he could not stand alone.

I must retract my earlier statement that I received no unsolicited information from the doctors. One morning very early I received a phone call from the neurosurgeon warning me not to worry, but Ted had fallen from the bed when the nurse's head was turned. "Very embarrassing," he said. "Don't be alarmed by the bandages and black eyes. We had to take ten stitches in his forehead. He'll be all right."

Shortly after that, after a bedside visit, the surgeon suggested to me that he call a psychiatrist because Ted seemed to be depressed: he had told one of the nurses that he saw no point in living and wished he were dead. It seemed to me a perfectly logical attitude. Who wouldn't want to die rather than lie there with a bandaged head, an oozing opening in his throat, and an infected hole in his stomach, unable to talk or walk. To me it was a sign of mental health to want to escape from all that. It did tell us, however, that we had to double our efforts to reassure him that he was loved by many people in addition to his family, that we needed and wanted him to continue to be among us, and that we would do all we could to help him get stronger.

I remember vividly an evening I spent with friends just before the end of Ted's hospitalization. When I came home that night I recorded my shock at their bickering at the dinner table when they recounted a story of their travels:

"No, it wasn't Wednesday we were there. It was Thursday..."

"You're wrong. I am sure it was a Wednesday."

"I know it was a Thursday because..." (voices rising).

How could I tell them how precious was the time they were wasting. They had each other, alive and well and walking. Then I quickly realized that a year ago Ted and

I, too, would probably have sounded like bickerers to others. I should have reminded us, then, as I wanted to say to my friends that night, that Thornton Wilder's Emily in *Our Town* spoke to our condition: "Do any human beings ever realize life while they live it?—every, every minute?"

As soon as Ted was moved onto "the floor," conversations began with the hospital social worker about his future. She had already begun to arrange for him to be transferred to Jefferson House, a skilled nursing facility in Newington a little over a mile from our home.

The potential expenses she outlined for his care there were overwhelming. Medicare would pay for the first ninety days *if* Ted were receiving care that only a registered nurse could administer. But the minute the gastrostomy tube was out, Medicare would not cover the expenses of ninety dollars a day. The qualifications for Medicaid (welfare) were so gloomy that I was depressed for days just contemplating them. "After you have used all your savings, your investments, and your retirement funds, you will still be able to keep your house," said the social worker, brightly. Keep it on what? What was I to use to pay for fuel, lights, and food?

Suddenly, on a very hopeless day, I remembered Norman Cousins again. In *The Anatomy of an Illness,* he had decided to move from the hospital to a hotel room so he could take his treatment into his own hands. If Ted were not incontinent, if he could learn to transfer from the bed to the wheelchair, I could take care of him at home. That long path in the wheelchair was becoming a near reality, and it seemed the logical, almost happy choice when Medicare payments would run out at the nursing home.

CHAPTER IV

New Horizons: The Skilled Nursing Facility

*I stepped from Plank to Plank
A slow and cautious way
The Stars about my Head I felt
About my Feet the Sea.*

*I knew not but the next
Would be my final inch—
This gave me that precarious Gait
Some call Experience.*

—*Emily Dickinson*

The bright sun on November 19 was a pale rival to our dispositions as we packed Ted, his plants, his cards, his air mattress, his turquoise plastic washbowls, and his daffodil-yellow urinals into the ambulance and moved to Jefferson House. During those days at the hospital when I had complained about his wrists being tied up and his being poked, prodded, and confined, a doctor friend had said, "Don't worry, he'll never remember *any* of this." How right she was. His memory did not begin again until he was in "Jeff House." The sight of eleven-year-old Kayden stringing large, decorated letters that spelled "Grandpa" across the wall of his room is his first memory since the night two months before when he was found by the policeman.

The nursing home experience is one shared by many people these days. Almost everyone my age has had friends or relatives involved in it, but it is not often written about with sympathy and understanding. I am quite sure I cannot, either, for one's expectations about the care one's "loved one" should receive and what happens in actuality are quite different.

On most days, I was in awe of the patience and kindness most of the staff exhibited under incredibly trying days and nights—cleaning wet and soiled beds; enduring the monotonous, unending call of "Nurse, Nurse"; spending long hours with those who were so disoriented that there could be no communication or, indeed, any hope of recuperation.

On other days, I would fret about the infrequency of the exercise Ted was getting; the overcooked, unpalatable food; and the long delays in answering a bell for help in getting to the bathroom. We were fortunate he could be in a beautiful, sunny, single room where Kayden and Bryn could decorate his walls with pictures and signs, and where we could try to arouse his interest in basketball games on his own television without having to contend with a roommate's soap operas. Because his tracheotomy had just been closed and was healing, talking with him was discouraging to visitors who found unfamiliar one-way conversations awkward and unsatisfying. I know now, however, how much those visits meant to him, for he remembers every person who came to see him in those long winter months.

For me, being able to drive the short distance to the nursing home, to find free parking places always available, and to have unlimited visiting time was a huge relief. My days fit into a rhythmical, predictable pattern quite different from the "hecticity" of the hospital. Predictable, that is, until the day of the blizzard in February when snow piled so high against both the front and back doors of our house that there was no way they could be opened. I was a prisoner inside until I discovered I could open a front window onto the porch. Cross-country skis in hand, I fell out of the window into a snow drift and proceeded to ski down the middle of Main Street to Jeff House. No one had expected any visitors that day, not even family.

My hours with Ted were punctuated with interesting bits of conversation, which I recorded in the journal.

"Ellen, get me out of here before they take me to the booby hatch. Get on the stick!"

"Ted," I laughed, "you *are* off your rocker if you think I'd let them take you to the booby hatch."

One day when I was reading Christmas cards aloud to him, he complained, "My ears don't have any attention span."

When friends visited, and many came, we always took the opportunity to walk Ted up and down the hall, supporting him on each side. The nurses were impressed when a Quaker friend who was a well-known television commentator on a local station came Sunday mornings to see Ted. He patiently helped Ted learn to speak more slowly and pronounce his words more clearly.

Twice during those three months, we brought Ted home for short visits. Our family usually celebrated Christmas day at Karen's house, but since we decided that that would be a little too chaotic for Ted's first trip away, we brought him home for the first time four days after Christmas, while Marcia was still here. We had lunch, sat in front of the fire, and listened to familiar records. He was not able to speak for awhile, but when we handed him a piece of paper and pencil, he wrote, laboriously, "Home, sweet home."

HOME   SWEET   HOME

Sometimes he was very feisty! One day I began a routine to test his awareness: "What town is this? What day is this? What month is this?" He raised his voice in exasperation. "Stop asking me those questions. I don't *care* what month it is! Karen does that all the time and it drives me batty."

"We're only doing what the book says," I said timidly.

"Throw out that book. *Bury* it!" he exclaimed.

We rejoiced at every sign of sustained interest. When he watched the Superbowl game all the way through, we cheered for him as well as for the Redskins—both won!

November, December, January. I think I was actually aware at the time that, in a way and for a brief time, I had the best of both worlds. Ted was being cared for twenty-four hours a day and was getting stronger. I had free hours to cross-country ski in the forests of the nearby reservoir, to go to plays and concerts in Hartford and New Haven, and to enjoy many dinners and evenings with generous, caring friends. That was an interim I was not to have again, and I appreciated it, but it was also not one I would want to repeat. Not a day passed when I did not look forward to having Ted home.

In anticipation of that time, we helped him walk down the hall using a walker, though it became evident that his impaired balance made it impossible for him to use it without assistance. He also needed help to transfer from the bed to the wheelchair, but once in it, he could explore the halls outside his room. At the nurse's suggestion, he began to wheel himself to the weekly meetings of the Stroke Club in the community room on his floor. It was at the first such meeting that he discovered what was wrong with him. He didn't know he had had a stroke, though many times in the hospital we had described the hemorrhage and the damage it had caused and thought

New Horizons

he understood us. He seemed more content, now that he could identify his problem, and he became interested in talking with others to compare their experiences and feelings with his own.

The date when he could come home was uncertain because of our precarious situation with Medicare. If the nurses withdrew Ted's gastrostomy tube, the payments would cease; and if they did not withdraw it, we could not know if he could take enough nourishment by mouth to enable him to survive at home!

Food was a bone of contention. We were all anxious for Ted to eat as much as possible and did not hide our disappointment when he sent back trays of food he had barely tasted. On one occasion, when I reminded him he needed to eat more so he would be strong enough to come home, he barked, "Roll the bed down. I can take your sermon lying down as well as sitting up!"

His days of crossness were rare, however. Once when I came in late after skiing all day, he said, "Oh, you're here. I thought you weren't coming. I tried to be strong, but I cried a lot."

In early February, after sessions with a psychologist who reported that Ted and I seemed to realize the problems awaiting us at home and would be able to cope with them, a conference was called with the nurses, social workers, physical and speech therapists, and the family doctor who was then caring for Ted. It was agreed that on the 24th of that month, Ted could leave Jefferson House. That was day 90 on the Medicare books.

Those February days were filled with preparations on the home front. Having bought a new station wagon in January with wheelchair space in mind, I now bought a second wheelchair, which would remain in the car. It proved a very wise investment. A carpenter installed handrails on the front and back porches, over the bathtub, and along the outside of the house. I purchased a bathtub bench and installed a frame around the toilet for support. I arranged an intercom system between Ted's downstairs bedroom and my upstairs bedroom, and ordered a cordless phone so he would not be disturbed by incessant ringing if I were out in the yard. I sewed patches of Velcro on large bathtowels to use for bibs and ordered shirts and trousers that fasten with Velcro.

The actual day of departure from Jeff House was a bit of a letdown. What to us was the end of a three-month pattern of daily contact, telephone calls, conferences, anxiety shared, and progress celebrated was just another routine signing-out for members of the staff, who gave us a casual wave and a couple of good-byes, and then turned down the hall to answer the ever-frantic cries of "Nurse, Nurse!"

Ted's arrival at home was undramatic, also. He immediately snuggled into his own bed, smiled at the daffodils on the table beside it, and fell sound asleep.

CHAPTER V

A New and Different Daily Life

Forever-is composed of Nows-
'Tis not a different time-
—Emily Dickinson

The next day, I had to figure out how to maneuver him from the bed into the wheelchair, from the wheelchair into the bathroom and onto the toilet. I also had to figure out how to wash him, shave him, see that he got his teeth brushed, get him dressed, clean up a soiled bed from top to bottom, and prepare a simple meal that I hoped he would not reject completely. That night, as I sat on the floor and untied his shoes, I thought that if I could survive that day I could survive anything, but I also had the sinking feeling that I could never leave the house again.

I remember the impact of that moment very well. In trying to balance the joy of having Ted home and the hard realities of a suddenly new and different daily life, I found myself repeating Emily Dickinson once more:

> *For each ecstatic instant*
> *We must an anguish pay*
> *In keen and quivering ratio*
> *To the ecstasy.*

The very next day I decided to eliminate what I saw as a threat of imprisonment. While Ted was napping, I visited a widowed neighbor two doors away to see if she would consider sitting in the house if Ted were asleep and I needed to be away. A perfect arrangement resulted: I paid her a rather large check in advance and then simply used up the hours as I needed her. It was a good investment for her; and her gentle, kind presence helped me feel very secure when I wanted to attend my regular Writers Group or Book Club, or have an evening out.

The trapped feeling disappeared very soon as I also discovered I could take Ted to movies, concerts, and plays without too much difficulty. We became very grateful for all evidences of the successful lobbyists for the handicapped, and we soon learned to resent unhandicapped people who take advantage of handicapped parking areas.

As soon as Ted came home, Medicare provided a succession of helpers from an organization of "healthproviders." The first physical therapist was a recent high school graduate, a robust young man who hesitantly tried to help Ted walk with a walker. On the day of his second session, Ted showed his orientation to the New Deal by saying to me at breakfast, "I better get through here in a hurry. That W.P.A. fella is coming this morning."

The "W.P.A." fellow did not last long, however, and a very pregnant young girl took his place. At the same time, a housekeeper was provided, four hours a day, five days a week. She was specifically instructed to do things for Ted only—no housework, lunches, cleaning, etc. I soon began to long for the day I could take over rather than fret about her sitting idle at the kitchen table for two hours after she had finished her limited duties.

An occupational therapist helped Ted learn to transfer himself from the bed to the wheelchair and from the wheelchair to the toilet—both great accomplishments. A speech therapist worked mostly with pronunciation of

A New and Different Daily Life

words. The third physical therapist who came was a very attractive, helpful person whom Ted liked very much, and who walked him from the bedroom to the living room with the walker once a week. But all these services ceased when Medicare decided Ted had reached a plateau and would not improve at a rate their guidelines said would qualify us for home care. This happened about two months after his return from Jeff House.

When our doctor at Kaiser learned about it, he immediately arranged for us to visit the Easter Seal Rehabilitation Center in Hartford for physical and speech therapy twice a week, paid for by Kaiser. There, Ted practiced walking with a quad-cane, assisted by someone on one side, and speech exercises improved his talking. The pitch of his voice was still a problem, however. One day after speech therapy, Ted explained, "When I get too involved emotionally, my voice goes up high. It got so high today when she had me reading 'The Gettysburg Address' that we had to switch to *Leaves of Grass.*"

His greatest concern during all this time was that he could not read. For five years before the stroke, a cataract in his right eye had limited his vision; now, the stroke had affected the vision in his left eye, as well. With his glasses off or on, he saw double.

For years, Ted had read according to a unique pattern, which he devised for himself but which he has steadfastly refused to call a hobby, saying he doesn't believe in such a thing. On the first Sunday of each month, he determined which best-seller had been on the *New York Times* Book Review Best Seller List for the most number of weeks. He did the fiction list in odd months and the nonfiction list in even months. He put this book on his list, bought it (by now it was usually in paperback), and added it to the row on the top of a special bookshelf in his study where it joined books from his other three categories: new books (usually gifts), books from our own bookshelves (he was systematically reading them one by one and then disposing of them unless I objected), and books from the French Book-of-the-Month Club, which he had belonged to ever since we lived in France for a while twenty-five years ago. Each day he read a certain number of pages in one book in each category, the amount of reading being determined by the days it would take to finish the book in one month. He started bestsellers in the first week of the month, new books the second week, French books the third week, and our bookshelf books the fourth week. You can imagine, then, his despair at being deprived of this stimulating, enlightening ritual.

Knowing how important improved vision would be to him, we had arranged for a cataract operation even before he left Jefferson House. His lens implant in April was a successful operation that enabled him after a few months to read, albeit slowly and tediously, with his right eye. Since, for all practical purposes, he had been using only one eye for several years anyway, the lack of binocular vision did not bother him. He has found that, if he wears a patch on his left eye, he can now read quite well with his right eye, though he constantly regrets not being able to read as easily and swiftly as he used to. This has slowed down his reading ritual but has not changed it in any other way. I smiled the day I discovered Erma Bombeck and Barbara Tuchman taking their places beside each other on his bookshelf.

His unpatched eye created a moment of terror for us one day when we returned from a day at Newport, R.I. As I wheeled Ted into the house, he exclaimed, "Everything is red, bright red. I can't see anything the way it should be. It's red, red, red." He stayed in bed all the next day to see if the situation would change. Things began to turn a lighter shade of red, and by the third day, they were a faint pink. Both of us assumed he had had a hemorrhage in his eye, behind the lens implant, and we were glad we had an appointment at Kaiser that Monday.

Our relief was immediate when the optometrist explained that the plastic lens inserted in the cataract operation does not absorb the rays of the sun as a natural lens does. "Daylong bright sunlight exhausted the blue-sensitive cones and rods and allowed the red rods to be overly stimulated." Sunglasses were advised.

On that same visit we asked our regular doctor about a large black-and-blue bruise that had suddenly appeared on Ted's arm. We had assumed, also, that it was a hemorrhage, and Ted had remarked, "If that had been in my brain, I'd be dead now."

"No connection with the artery that hemorrhaged in your brain," explained the doctor. "This happens often in older people and especially in hot weather. The veins are very near the surface; capillaries break and spread. No connection with your stroke." We decided on the way home that Kaiser should adopt our local jeweler's motto: Peace of Mind Guaranteed.

My journal ended the day Ted came home, but I keep finding small pieces of paper and backs of envelopes on which I wrote snatches of his conversation or comments.

In August, my sister from Ohio came to stay with Ted so that I could go to the Martin Luther King anniversary demonstration in Washington. She was amused by Ted's sense of humor and, as an example, reported his response to a farmer-neighbor of hers who had told her that, in the spring, he always sat on a piece of his land to figure out when it was dry enough to plant his crops.

"I guess that's the ass-id test," commented Ted.

When I urged him to shave right after breakfast, he explained, "No, I'm not going to shave until after my nap. My whiskers grow while I sleep."

When he saw the package from which I'd taken a cupcake, he said scornfully, "If I'd known it was called 'Twinkie,' I wouldn't have eaten it!"

And one night he pointed to a hole a moth had eaten in his sweater.

"Is it corrupted then?" I asked.

"No," he immediately replied. "No rust. Just moths."

On the occasions when I took him in the car while I shopped, I often asked him to make some sociological observations while I was in the store. Once when I emerged, my arms filled with groceries, he reported, "My survey tells me that women who wear men's pants should also wear men's shoes. And also, that food stores must be very cleverly arranged because not one person comes out with just one thing."

In summer, noticing how many people seem to carry a can of some kind to drink from as they walk along, he opined that nobody drinks unflavored water anymore. And he is convinced that the three things that have caused the downfall of the young, and therefore of civilization, are television, the computer, and catsup.

His vocabulary is sometimes startling. One time when I referred to a trip we had taken the summer before, he quickly observed, "That was before your paramour went berserk."

During a winter storm, I found Ted sitting in his wheelchair looking out the window at the falling snow and murmuring,

> *The snow had begun in the gloaming*
> *And busily all the night*

A New and Different Daily Life

Had been heaping the field and highway
With a silence deep and white....

For days he kept repeating these words, trying to remember the rest of the four verses and the author of this poem he had memorized when he was eleven years old. He searched his collections of Longfellow, Emerson, and Whittier to no avail. Finally, at the suggestion of one of his colleagues, a professor of English, we found the poem "The First Snowfall" in a James Russell Lowell collection. We also discovered the reason Ted's teacher had had her pupils learn only the first four verses: she probably wanted to protect her sixth graders from the tragic death of a child and the accompanying theology in the last four verses.

Another fragment that kept nagging at Ted was

When I consider how my light is spent
Ere half my days, in this dark world and wide,...

He was able to complete Milton's sonnet "On His Blindness" as soon as he took down Mark van Doren's *Anthology of World Poetry* from our bookshelf.

I realize in writing these bits of conversation that they must not seem very unusual to anyone else, but I seized upon any flash of humor or insight or memory as a sign that Ted's "superosity was segatiating," a phrase my grandfather used to describe one's state of well-being and which was a steadfast criterion in our family's own particular Bureau of Standards.

CHAPTER VI

The Nitty-Gritty

To make Routine a Stimulus
Remember it can cease–
Capacity to Terminate
Is a Specific Grace–
   —*Emily Dickinson*

Do not be deceived by my writing only about smiles, good humor, and poems. The nitty-gritty is very real, and my list of complaints, though not long, is a daily reminder of all the distractions, interruptions, frustration, and impatience.

It begins with a vision of sitting down at dinnertime to a plate of fresh asparagus, cooked just right, new potatoes nestling in the hot, pink juice of a steak from the broiler, and Ted backing away from the table, announcing, "I want to go to the toilet." Though he can manage this by himself, I know that by helping him we shall both be able to enjoy a good meal sooner, but I wonder why the trip couldn't have been anticipated before the meal!

Another constant irritation is that I expect him to know that he should release the brakes on his wheelchair whenever I get ready to push it. Any irritation or annoyance in my "Release, Ted, please" provokes a much larger annoyance in his "How should *I* know what you want?"

I often want demanding tones to be mitigated by a "please" or "thank you," which he uses without fail with

The Nitty-Gritty

strangers or friends, but I realize that with me they would need to be so constant they would surely lose their meaning.

His pain is not the same as other people's pain, either: it is on a different scale. About once a week I hear a cry from the bedroom—an anguished, desperate call. On the way to answer it, I rehearse the phone number for the ambulance, decide how to get in touch with Karen and Marcia, and begin to plan the memorial service, but when I arrive at the bedside, "I have this rough place on my fingernail. Could you hand me the clippers?"

The daily routines carry their own kind of weariness. I remember the moment I realized the enormous tasks that stretched ahead for me: I would carry out every ounce of trash that ever accumulated in our house; I would lug every load of firewood that would ever be carried to our fireplace; I would wash every dish that was ever dirty; I would change every fuse that would ever blow; I would mow down every blade of grass that pushed its way up in our lawn. It struck me then that I had all the disadvantages of being single and none of its advantages (and it seems to me there are several, contrary to the opinions of some of my unwed friends).

There is one strange advantage in my new situation, however, that I must not forget to mention. I suddenly realized one day how much time and psychological energy I was saving by not worrying about why Ted was not doing what I thought he ought to be doing. It is a common problem among those of us who are retired, and I expect as the leaders of the National Organization for Women grow older, they will address it. A man retires to sit and read and enjoy his unplanned hours. A woman does not retire from grocery shopping, preparing meals, or cleaning house. In addition, her mind is not so busy that it cannot see walls to be painted, remodeling that might be done, yards that could be relandscaped. To be released from making all those futile, unacceptable suggestions to the retired partner relieves one of an immense amount of fretting.

Some of that released energy will now be spent in praise of an object without which we could never have survived the months and years since Ted's stroke. It is a yellow plastic rectangle, with a handle, which narrows at one end to a round opening. It is called a urinal. The presence of this indispensable utensil has meant no nighttime trips to the bathroom, no terrible anxieties on long automobile rides, and no problems in strange motels or hotel bedrooms.

No problems, maybe, but some mighty funny moments—funny, at least, in retrospect. I will never forget the night we went camping with nine other couples near Tanglewood, the music festival center in Lenox, Mass. It had rained all day, and our usual picnic on the lawn was of necessity spread out on a picnic table under a shed-roof near the entrance to the festival grounds. I should have expected it, but I didn't. The moment the tortellini salad, French baguettes, wine, and piles of fresh fruit were ready on the table, while the rain came down in torrents just outside, from Ted came "I want to go to the toilet." There was nothing to do but push the wheelchair down the flooded pathway into a drenched corner of the woods and brush, and struggle to hold an umbrella over the two of us while I produced the handy yellow rectangle. It had been resting in a blue-and-white tote bag bearing the name of a leading Quaker publication, *The Friends Journal*. In memory of some faraway Swedish ancestors of Ted's, I immediately rechristened the bag "The Friends Yur'nal."

The Nitty-Gritty

My celebration of the urinal is equaled by my enthusiasm for the other aspect of elimination. I have always maintained that the bathroom is the most holy space in all of Christendom, for many more prayers are offered there than in any cathedral, church, or temple (prayers, for example, that one *is,* or just as fervently, *isn't* menstruating). In our case, supplications are for a regular, normal bowel movement. For me, it is in this small room that an unparalleled reverence manifests itself: I am in constant awe of the high-tech ability of the human body as it programs the proper distribution of proteins, carbohydrates, minerals, vitamins, and fiber to produce a remarkable printout of growth, strength, energy, and vitality. The resultant efficient, healthy disposal of waste is a sign that this magnificent machine is functioning at its best and is cause for high praise. The painful and disastrous results when there is a malfunction are dreadful enough to warrant the faithful following of any regimen necessary to guarantee success.

This is a phenomenon that is with us as children, as parents, and when, as older citizens, we become acutely aware of the full circle of life. One day I found myself exclaiming "Good for *you!*" in the holy of holies. The neighbors could hear me laughing.

Having certain bodily functions under control makes it possible to be much more mobile, allowing us not only to enjoy events in Hartford, New Haven, Boston, or New York, but also to travel much longer distances. In fact, journeying by air becomes almost more convenient than getting to local destinations. The concern of the airlines' personnel for their wheelchair passengers makes a trip pleasant instead of dreadful.

In August, six months after Ted's return home, we flew to the University of Wisconsin in Madison so he could attend a board meeting of the Alexander Meiklejohn Experimental College Foundation and a seminar sponsored by alumni of the college. At that time we checked Ted's wheelchair through to Madison and were escorted to and from planes in the airline's wheelchairs, attendants carrying Ted in a special chair to and from his plane seat.

When we attended the board meeting the next year, Ted was able to walk onto the plane with assistance. Since the car we rented in Madison was a hatchback, our wheelchair could fit into it conveniently when we traveled.

One of our side trips included a visit with Ted's cousin near Green Bay. There Ted learned great adaptability, for her house had no downstairs bathroom or bedroom. He proved quite adept at pulling himself upstairs along the railing and coming downstairs, rumpwise, the way we women were advised to do, postpregnancy, forty or fifty years ago!

At Florida's Disneyworld in January 1984, we found a real haven for the handicapped; whenever we approached a long waiting line at Epcot Center, a guide motioned us to the exit of the exhibit, where we were admitted within a few minutes and were adroitly helped into a moving car or wobbly boat, leaving our wheelchair at the starting point.

Later that year we attended an Elderhostel in Flagstaff, Ariz., where many volunteers among our fellow "students" took turns pushing Ted's wheelchair, stowing it in the luggage space of the bus that took us to the campus each day, and helping when I tried to balance two trays on my arm in the cafeteria line. At Northern Arizona University we studied the history of the Anasazi and visited ruins of their pueblos, and we got a close-up view

The Nitty-Gritty

of the moon at the Lowell Observatory. When we took a field trip to the Grand Canyon, I was able to push Ted along the smooth asphalt path near the rim, where we could read the graph of centuries on the walls of that gray-purple-blue-pink gash in the earth.

After Ted's Meiklejohn Foundation board meeting in California in 1985, we flew north to visit in Oregon and Washington. We discovered that, from Portland to Seattle, we could take a train that has a special car to accommodate wheelchairs, so we went by rail for that short distance. We rolled up a ramp; established ourselves in spacious, comfortable seats; and thoroughly enjoyed the views from our wide, low windows as we traveled along the shore of Puget Sound.

I will pass along a bit of advice to others traveling as we do: I always wear a suit with large pockets into which I put rolls of dollar bills at the start of each trip. If anyone even smiles at me he is apt to get a bill thrust in his hand, and the porters, especially the one who wheeled Ted into the men's room at O'Hare airport, receive several peels from the roll.

When a porter isn't available, I stand near the men's room and try to judge which man entering would not mind taking Ted in. I can still see the relief on one woman's face in Florida when her husband finally emerged after twenty minutes, pushing Ted's wheelchair. Had I only known which woman was the wife, I could have explained what errand of mercy was delaying her husband.

Of course, there are times that are unpleasant, irritating, and discouraging while traveling, just as there are at home; but they are easily offset by the stimulation that comes from new scenery and gracious friends and relatives. Of our life in general, I can confidently say that my list of "be grateful fors" is longer than my list of complaints: Ted is not paralyzed, he is not blind, he is not deaf, he can feed himself, he sleeps well, and he has not had any pain. Most of all, he can think and remember and speak.

If I am ever tempted to forget this longer list and dwell on the annoyances and frustrations, all I have to do is ask myself, "What must it be like for Ted?" What must it be like to be unable to get up out of a wheelchair and get something you want from a top shelf; what must it be like to know you can't get in the car and drive to town to take your suit to the cleaners because, even if you could drive, you couldn't get out of the car by yourself; what must it be like to know you can't drive your granddaughter to the birthday party of a friend? These are three incapabilities Ted has bemoaned recently, and many more desires, I know, are unexpressed.

One of his worst frustrations must be not being able to speak as well as he used to. He was a prize-winning debater in high school; in fact, one girl in his senior class had written in his yearbook, "I'm pretty certain that ten years from now you'll be one of the leading orators in our country." How painful it must be to speak so slowly that the normal give and take in a conversation is halted and usually followed by a request to repeat his contribution.

Those with whom he speaks must pay special attention, listen more carefully, and be very, very patient. For a witty conversationalist who used to hold forth on many pet, controversial ideas, this must be very frustrating, and I admit parties are less colorful when Ted is not able to proclaim, when appropriate, "The automobile has *got* to *go!*" and other startling maxims. He is known as the most optimistic pessimist his friends have ever met, and we all miss the insights from that particular perspective

The Nitty-Gritty

when we are too impatient to absorb his halting contributions. He was also referred to by his colleagues, after heated arguments, as the most militant pacifist they knew. Now they find the adjective subdued, but the noun has not changed; he is still their ethical guru.

Some of us are guilty, sometimes, of assuming that a person who is hard to understand in speech is also somewhat retarded. An example of the effect of this liaison in the public mind occurs when someone sees Ted in a wheelchair and automatically raises his voice to a near shout, or begins to use simple words and phrases he would use with a child. Ted is a good sport about accepting all this, but for him, whose mind races so far ahead of his words, it must be a painful experience to be asked so often to repeat what he has said, or, worse still, to be left to sit alone in the corner of the room because he cannot keep up with the chatter of others.

This change in the ability to communicate, as well as his physical limitations, does cause moments of despondence, of course, and they are very painful for both of us. "It would have been better for you, for me, and for everyone if I had died that night." Or once, when I described how much freer he was from illnesses now than when he was five years old, he said wistfully, "But when I was five years old I could walk."

Most of the time, however, Ted has accepted the irrevocable change in his life with little complaining. I admire tremendously his way of adjusting, his unbelievably good spirits, and his amazing sense of humor. His ability to live in the present, his refusal to dwell on what might have been or to dread what may be, has stood him in good stead these months. Alexander Meiklejohn's previously quoted statement applies: "Intelligence...is readiness for any human situation; it is the power, wherever one goes, of being able to see, in any set of circumstances, the best response which a human being can make to those circumstances."

Ted's days now are filled with a rather quiet routine, punctuated with concerts, plays, movies, dinners with family and friends, his regular set-back parties, and Quaker meetings. The routine consists of starting the day with basic physical and speech exercises recommended by his therapists, reading the newspaper, napping, awaiting the arrival of the day's mail, lunch, and, after a second nap, reading from his four books, concurrently, and listening to the incredibly fine Talking Books for the Blind or Physically Handicapped from the state library. He has listened to four Dickens's novels, but one of his orders was a bit more eclectic: Ken Follett's *On Wings of Eagles,* C. Wright Mills's *The Power Elite,* Richard Henry Dana's *Two Years Before the Mast,* and James Kahn's *Star Wars: Return of the Jedi.* I mustn't forget the many hours spent listening to the Red Sox baseball games on the radio or watching football games on television, especially when a Green Bay Packers game is telecast. And always there is the evening news.

On Fridays the routine is broken by a pattern that Ted has agreed to, reluctantly, so I will have some time for myself. He spends that day in the nearby Adult Day Care Center (see chap. 9). Sometimes the participants are there for some of the same reasons that such centers exist for very "junior" citizens: no one is at home during the day, or respite is needed for parents or caregivers from full-time obligations. I fit into the latter category: the uninterrupted few hours I have on Fridays are greatly treasured.

Unplanned time is indeed a luxury. After years of hectic schedules, demanding deadlines, and wanting to

The Nitty-Gritty

be where I was not, I found in Kurt Vonnegut's *Deadeye Dick* the word to fit a philosophy that was beginning to emerge when I retired from my job in public relations at a local college:

> We all see our lives as stories, it seems to me. . . . If a person survives an ordinary span of sixty years or more, there is every chance that his or her life as a shapely story has ended, and all that remains to be experienced is epilogue. . . . Some people . . . find inhabiting an epilogue . . . uncongenial.

Some find, as I have, that the epilogue can be the best part of a life.

I don't think my interpretation of this "epilogue" is the same one Vonnegut intended in his novel, but to me, who always found the epilogue the best part of any book, the word has particular meaning. For the same reasons I like that section after the last chapter, I like this time to evaluate, to pull together loose ends, to see a pattern in the fabric of the past. In the very large implications, it means coming to terms not only with life but also with death, a not-to-be-feared, very-appropriate-in-the-scheme-of-things occasion.

There is a great release when the stress of having to produce and achieve disappears, and one's time is given over to extracting from each moment a distillate that is rich and heady. The accumulation of *things* becomes obscene, and the frantic race from one event to another slows down—not to a halt, to be sure, but to a healthy, selective pace, which enables us to savor what we have chosen.

Savor is the word: "To impart flavor, scent, or a distinctive quality to." We savor friendships, making as many opportunities as possible to be with friends, spontaneously, informally. Amid the frustrations, disappointments, and impatient times, I find intense pleasure in small events: reading, in a hammock, all the *New Yorker* on the day it arrives; enjoying a picnic lunch in the backyard under the watchful gaze of a border of black-eyed Susans; cheering with a daughter at a political rally; returning my granddaughter's teasing laugh. Most of all, I rejoice when I come into the kitchen for the first time in the morning and find Ted in his wheelchair, fully dressed, reading the *Courant*. I am overwhelmed when he looks up and says with such quiet warmth, "Hello, Ellen."

In my mind's eye flashes the long list of "Ted's Achievements," which we keep on the bulletin board: from small tasks, such as buttering his own toast, pouring cream on his cereal, putting toothpaste on his toothbrush, clipping his own toenails, and washing his hair, to larger tasks, such as getting on and off the toilet from the wheelchair, and bathing and dressing himself. It was a happy coincidence that he learned that he could stay in the house alone just at the time our neighbor-sitter moved away. He had been terrified by the idea of fire, but now he has enough confidence to know he could crawl to a door or climb out his first-floor window if he had to. One of his greatest accomplishments was being able to ride with Marcia to Philadelphia to spend four days with her. He could do this because he was strong enough to walk with her support and thus get about in her small row house without his wheelchair.

When they came back to Connecticut after that trip, we gathered the family together for a picture to be taken on the occasion of our forty-fifth wedding anniversary. The faces in that photo are happy ones, as were those in the picture Bryn took the night before Ted's stroke. Not one anguished hour in the intervening years has been

The Nitty-Gritty

forgotten, but neither have the hours of concerned love, support, and encouragement from friends, from relatives, and from each other.

We find ourselves in the midst of the miracles that William Blake wrote about and that, for me, describe our epilogue.

> *To see a World in a Grain of Sand*
> *And a Heaven in a Wild Flower,*
> *Hold Infinity in the palm of your hand*
> *And Eternity in an hour.*

In September, exactly three years after his stroke, Ted rode with the family to Sullivan Stadium in Foxboro, Mass., to see his beloved Green Bay Packers play the Patriots!

"I got a neat picture of Grandpa buying hot dogs," boasted Bryn.

CHAPTER VII

"The Story of a Stroke"

This is my letter to the World....
—Emily Dickinson

The preceding chapters appeared, with some modifications, in an article entitled "The Story of a Stroke," which was published in *Northeast,* the Sunday magazine of the *Hartford Courant,* on October 13, 1985.

I had been working on the story for a couple of years, basing parts of it on the journal I kept when Ted was in the hospital and the nursing home, in order to have something to read at our monthly Writers Group meetings. For forty years we have met, and I didn't want to risk being out of good standing by being unproductive. After hearing several of my short pieces, the group encouraged me to put them together in an article that would tell the story of our three years since Ted's stroke.

When I finished a first draft, I decided I had better show it to Ted. I helped him climb the stairs to our beautiful, bright sunroom and seated him in the big, comfortable reclining chair. I handed it to him with some trepidation, wondering how he would feel about a story in which he was the main character. It took him more than an hour to read the manuscript. My heart was in my throat—how would he respond? He sat quietly for a moment after he put it down and then said, brokenly,

"The Story of a Stroke"

"It's good. It made me cry. Now you better get me to the bathroom. I don't want to get this chair wet."

The two members of our Writers Group who had written for *Northeast* urged me to send it there. The editor who accepted it and his associates were extremely helpful in suggesting cuts and changes so it would fit into their available space. I cannot say enough in praise of their expertise, their patience, their kindness, and their professionalism.

On that rainy October Sunday when the article appeared, I was very nervous. Would anyone take time to read it? Would anyone relate to our ups and downs? Was I too critical of the hospital or the nursing home? Would many who read it think it was maudlin? Was it too much exposure? Would we ever be able to walk down the aisle at the Symphony Concert without being stared at?

The first call that came that morning was a complete surprise.

"Hey, I just saw that article in the *Courant* magazine. Golly, that's just great. I sure liked the story. I really did. You know, Katharine Hepburn was on the cover of that magazine once, and now you. Golly!"

It was the young man who shovels snow from our driveway.

There were not many other calls that day—in fact, only two from people who had not known ahead of time the article was coming out. Brooding in front of the fire that evening and feeling a little let down, I remembered a footnote in my sociology textbook fifty years ago: a social scientist named Thomas proclaimed that every human being wishes for four things: security, new experience, recognition, and response. I expect there is a new vocabulary today to describe our needs and desires, but that evening the old-fashioned ones spoke to my condition. I said to myself: you are just like a child, wanting instant gratification. Look around you. Count what you've got! There I was, sitting in front of my fireplace, secure and comfortable in a warm home; I had had the shocking new experience of seeing my husband's and my faces, in full color, looking out from the cover of a magazine; inside that cover was a story recognized as valuable by a talented editor and his associates. Three out of four wishes fulfilled wasn't too bad, I realized. And the fourth, when you come right down to it, is pretty much of an ego trip.

But not entirely: I missed feedback, feeling incomplete until I knew if anyone else had had the same problems Ted and I had faced, if anyone else had identified with the yo-yo aspects of a tragedy.

Impatient me! In the next few days and weeks, my fourth wish was fulfilled a thousandfold! There were calls from friends as well as from strangers whose husbands or wives had had strokes and wanted to talk about them; from a lawyer who said the article helped her as she tried to encourage her former law professor who was suffering a deep depression after his stroke; from a neighbor: "Were we the bickerers?"; from a former student friend: "You probably didn't know, but I'm getting married soon. My fiance is a little older than I am. I gave him your story today and said that when he finishes it, I want it to be the jumping-off point for a discussion."

One day after the mail came, I put a dozen letters and cards on the table and said excitedly to Ted, "Look at all these letters from friends about our story!"

He acknowledged my remark with a brief nod of his head, reached for the University of Wisconsin Alumni Association Membership Directory, which had come in the same mail, and turned immediately to see if his name was spelled correctly. Well, I thought, each of us gets on a different bus for our own particular ego trip.

Some of the most touching communications were from Ted's former students; his eyes filled with tears as I read them aloud:

> At first, I was haunted by the face on the cover, but that totally made sense when I realized that twenty-two years have passed since I've been in his class. I don't expect him to remember me, as I was just one of the thousands of students that have passed through his door. However, I do want him to know that I certainly do remember him and I'm very happy to read that he's doing better. I would like him to know that in the two years I spent in his classes perhaps he did teach me something even better than history. I would like to think that I learned a bit about life and caring.

And another:

> There was a time when history meant the memorization of events and dates. In 1952-53, Dr. Paullin opened a new world for me and history became human and exciting! . . . I remember I "baby-sat" for your children one evening while you attended a college function. You were kind enough to allow my boyfriend to come also! . . . My husband died of a heart attack six years ago and I am disabled with lung disease so I understand . . . pain and frustration. Your story helps me personally to feel less alone with the struggle.

A student of thirty years ago wrote that she recognized her history professor's picture and wanted him to know how much she could identify with our story:

> My husband will never be as strong, as well, or as untiring as he was before his illness . . . but we are grateful for each day we have together. We are thankful for the times I nag him to get a haircut when we think of how we worried about his losing his hair when he was so sick. I listen with contentment to every snore instead of poking and saying "Turn on your side." . . . I thank you for reminding me of a time when I learned what loving is all about.

A colleague of Ted's wrote, "I was reminded of wisdom learned, and forgotten, along the way. My father took me to *Our Town* when I was twelve, and Emily's return on her birthday is as vivid as it was back then, but I needed reminding."

From a young philosophy professor we heard, "I plan to file the article for future reference, perhaps thirty years or so along life's path (if not sooner). In fact, I've already quoted a few lines to my wife by way of commenting on our own everyday challenges." And the health director in a nearby town wrote, "It should make physicians, nurses, and therapists more sensitive to the patient and family's point of view."

Others wrote honest, well-deserved criticisms from their points of view: nurses on the floor where Ted had spent those agonizing two months wondered why I hadn't remarked about all the good they had accomplished—after all, Ted was alive and well, so his care couldn't have been too bad. And a nursing home attendant, commenting on the paragraph about my disappointment in the casual farewells as we left for home after three months there, exclaimed, very justifiably, "What did she want? A brass band?" In rereading the article I realize I could rewrite those parts now, having more perspective and understanding of the pressures the nurses and doctors are subject to, but at the time I wrote out of my frustrations, my weariness, my worries. I hadn't given a very objective account of the many invaluable skills and services which Ted had benefited from and which I appreciate more and more every day.

Among the many letters sent to the *Courant* were several very discerning ones commenting on and differing with my remarks linking an adult day care center and a nursery school. I saw their point immediately and hope I have corrected that impression in chapter 9.

Two communications from complete strangers have resulted in new and valued friendships.

One came after the editor forwarded a letter from a young woman whose husband is suffering from Parkinson's disease. She had written a poem about it, reflecting on their vacation days at Cape Cod in their "storm-wrinkled cottage," the days when "the silent terror" began, and finally, the "mixmaster phrases that now amuse us." I called her immediately to express my appreciation for the poem. Since then, Joe and Deanie and Ted and I have gotten together every month for lunch to share unusual experiences with wheelchairs, new gadgets, old remedies, urinals, and menus, and to find humor and hope where we can.

One Saturday morning about a month after the article appeared, I got a call from Rockford, Ill. Tottie Johnson introduced herself, saying a Connecticut friend had sent her the story and she wanted me to know that she had lived through every word of it. Her husband, Hugh, a plastic surgeon, had had a stroke in 1980, and as she told me some of their experiences since then, I found myself laughing in spite of the seriousness of their situation.

"What do you do when Ted falls?" she asked.

"He doesn't fall," I replied.

"Well, you haven't *lived!*" she exclaimed, and described trying to help her two-hundred-pound husband, whose left side is paralyzed, maneuver himself to a chair and get himself off the floor.

"The worst thing I did recently was to pin him under the overhead garage door." I cringed as she described how the neighbors came to help her lift the door and drag Hugh, unharmed, from under it.

In a letter that followed our phone conversation, she told of the loyal support of their three children, of Hugh's wilderness camping trip with his son, of a trip to England with his daughter, of his regular swimming sessions after his initial post-stroke fear of the pool, and of many colorful incidents along the way. I wrote back, asking for any helpful or unusual "tips" she could send us.

The following week I got a letter full of stories both tragic and comic, but also with good, commonsense suggestions:

> I'll bet your Connecticut winters are as hard to get through as our Illinois ones. Overcoats are such a struggle that I made Hugh a poncho out of 2½ yards of very heavy 54" wool. I cut a slit for the head and bound that and the two rough edges with 1" green binding—many people ask if the garment came from Austria! Hugh copes easily with it—no front, no back, no right side, no wrong side.

Her letters since then have combined her superb sense of humor with practical ideas:

> A lot of dignity and self-esteem fly out the window with a stroke. It makes a grown man feel like a child when he has to ask someone to cut his meat. Hugh

was delighted when we found a special knife that cuts by a rocking rather than a sawing motion. The blade is shaped slightly like a scimitar."*

In another letter she wrote,

> You'd get a kick our of our recent confrontation. We were going out for lunch, and I had gone ahead to survey the situation in a local restaurant when I suddenly heard a siren. As I went back, mission accomplished, I was amazed to see Hugh on the ground, a crowd gathered, and an ambulance approaching. I could see that the fall had shaken but not hurt him, and so I said, "He's all right. He's my husband."
>
> "Are you sure?" said the policeman.
>
> "Sure that he's my husband? Of course I am!" I said indignantly.

Later, Tottie wrote about two problems that had begun to bother me, too.

> There's so much frustration and so much nagging in this situation. How many times have I said, "Get your left leg back, touch the chair seat with it." I can see that he's going to crash down if he isn't squarely in the seat. Would it be possible for people such as Hugh to work in groups so they could watch each other and profit? I just wish there could be someone else to criticize, suggest, and nag. It's so hard not to be constantly urging him *to do* or *not to do*!

In my mind I quickly devised a new service for some entrepreneur: "Nag, Inc.—professional scolding, reminding, plain-and-fancy nagging—hourly rates."

*Distributed by Fred C. Sammons, Box 32, Brookfield, Ill. 60153.

Once Tottie wrote seriously about a situation I face often:

> One thing I will never say to anyone, I hope, is "What can I do to help?" Instead, I'm going to say "I'm on my way to the store and would be glad to pick up something for you." Or "I'm going to the concert and would be glad to come by and pick you up." It's all these decisions that get me down! I just love it when we get picked up and dropped off, when there is someone *else* to park the car!

I smiled, remembering the strange sense of freedom I feel when someone else just pushes Ted's wheelchair for me. I know, however, how that wheelchair intimidates people, and they hesitate to offer rides to us, thinking we can't fit into their cars.

A few months later, Tottie wrote about "the little Rascal," a motorized vehicle that has made it possible for Hugh to get about town by himself, to go to the hospital for meetings, and in general to feel very independent. "We'll come by Newington on our way to Massachusetts where we're spending the summer and show you Hugh's three-wheeled wonder." They did just that and we enjoyed our time together immensely.

The friendship resulting from the article in *Northeast* has had such rich rewards for us! Tottie's letters far outnumber the other responses I've had, but going through all of them recently, I found another writer who made a profound impression on me again, as she had when I read her letter the first time. She is a friend, a Superior Court judge, and she wrote about her feelings in relation to the "epilogue" with which I concluded my article:

"The Story of a Stroke"

As I see my "epilogue" beginning just around the corner, I wonder, as so many of us do at this age, just what the script will contain if we are lucky enough to live long lives. Your account of Ted's stroke and the honest and touching and funny way you both saw your way through that chapter of your lives is something I will always remember. You don't make it sound easy, but you make it sound possible and infinitely rewarding, and maybe that is the way anything is in life that is worth having. I . . . sometimes get the feeling that all of my life so far has been preparation or training for something, I don't know what. Starting with the toilet training and the piano lessons and the education and the flossing—what are we getting ready for? I was beginning to think perhaps it was preparation for death with grace, but your article suggests that maybe it is preparation for the unexpected adventures of the Last Chapter of those of us lucky enough to survive to a good age. Somehow that seems a bit more satisfying to me.

After describing her mother's experiences in a nursing home, she added, "We always wish 'long life' to those we love, and I suppose the real test of faith . . . is acceptance of whatever comes along, with 'Why me?' the ultimately arrogant question."

Indeed, it is an arrogant question. Karen and I were contemplating it that first night as we sat in the ER waiting to see Ted.

"The only logical question is 'Why *not* me?'" said Karen, logically.

CHAPTER VIII

The Phenomenon of Support Groups

"This is Henry Beaulieu," said the energetic voice on the phone, "and I just want you to know that I really go along with you on that article you wrote in *Northeast* magazine. I've been through everything you talked about there. My wife had a stroke a few months before your husband did, and I am the one who cares for her every day and every night."

We talked about some of the circumstances of Bernadette's stroke, and at the end of the conversation Henry said, "Why don't you folks come to our Stroke Club meeting? We have a good group that gets together the second Tuesday of every month. Come to the Community Center in Wethersfield—I think you'll enjoy it."

Not being too enthusiastic about it, I murmured something about our time schedule and said we'd think about it. Somehow the idea of a group of people getting together, some in wheelchairs, some with walkers, many with canes, seemed to me an invitation to discouragement. How could such a group have a sociable afternoon when what they had in common was disability.

How wrong I was!

When we decided to attend our first meeting of the Stroke Club, it was a rainy day. As usual I had trouble manipulating the umbrella over Ted's head and pushing

The Phenomenon of Support Groups

the wheelchair up the ramp into the Community Center. Parked beside our car was a bus from a Connecticut town on the shore, about thirty miles away. Wheelchairs and walkers were being unloaded from it, and people were laughing and talking as they slowly made their way behind us.

Joan Haines, who had started this support group, made us feel welcome immediately, and we soon found ourselves at a table with Henry and his wife, Bernadette, exchanging stories and experiences. When everyone was settled, Joan presided over an informal program.

"Chappy, you said last month you were going to do something you haven't done since you had your stroke: write a letter to your cousin. Do you have it?"

Chappy hung his head, then said slowly, "Next time. I'll do it—next time."

Joan patted him on the back. "I'm sure you will."

Then she asked the group, "Anything new since last time that anyone wants to tell us about?"

"No, dammit," came a loud reply from a bearded man in a wheelchair at the back.

"Well, at least your voice is stronger, Peter." The group laughed.

Joan continued. "Today we have visitors from another Stroke Club, and we'd like to get to know each other. Let's just go around the room."

One by one the different stories came. One was told by a father whose young daughter is completely paralyzed and unable to speak. She was in tears, but he comforted her as he spoke and she became calm. The wife of a Chinese gentleman, formerly a professor at a local university, described the acupuncture treatments he is getting three times a week in New York. He nodded his head and smiled as she spoke. One man pointed out the window to his specially equipped van with a hoist, which lifts him, in his wheelchair, into the driver's place. "We can go anywhere," he said with confidence. "Next week we're off to Florida for a month." Our new friend, Henry, told of all the things he has learned taking care of his wife. "I bet I know how to put pantyhose on someone as well as any woman in this room!" he boasted.

And so on, around the circle: a tennis coach who had had to retire to care for his wife; a middle-aged woman who demonstrated how she gets around in her motorized scooter; a young man with a cane whose stroke had cut short a career in neurology. A twenty-four-year-old girl who had a stroke when she was eleven told us, "I like to write," and later she read one of her stories to the group. "I'm beginning to paint again," said a lovely gray-haired woman happily.

Some had evident paralysis; some had no paralysis but some speech problems. Some were aphasic, reaching for words that came out only with tremendous effort; the group patiently waited for their contributions.

The last man was from the visiting group. "Well, I tell you, there are some funny situations in this business." He began to chuckle. "I can't help laughing when I think about what happened to me this week. You see, my problem is my balance—I'm never very sure whether I have it or not. But I like to work in the garden, so I get out there whenever I can. This time when I was finished I stood up and suddenly I felt I was going to fall, so I hobbled over to a trash can that was near and sat on top of it. The lid wasn't on tight so as soon as I sat down the lid moved over and I fell in! My arms and my legs were sticking out and there I was—stuck in the trash can! Nobody was around, but I figured my wife would be home from work in about four hours and she'd probably find me."

The Phenomenon of Support Groups

We've attended Stroke Club ever since, finding a community of people who are making the best of what most of us would consider disastrous situations, with caregivers who are unendingly patient and kind. We have been surprised at the variety of the programs during the year. Members have made pies together, learned new exercises for the handicapped, taken part in a clown meeting where some became "performers," gone to the Ice Capades, and enjoyed a watermelon picnic at June Larson's farm. At one member's insistence, one meeting turned into a dance. With canes and wheelchairs people moved to the music. "I'm going to dance at my son's wedding next month!" exclaimed one man who had thought he would never be on a dance floor again. I have shown the color slides of our trips to China and the USSR at two of the programs, and found many in the group who have traveled widely. They have been encouraged to bring their slides for future programs.

The leader of the group, Joan Haines, is an attractive young nurse, whose husband is a veterinarian. His partner's wife, June Larson, an expert horsewoman all her life, suffered a stroke while taking her horses to a show and was hospitalized for weeks. (That is strange: why do we always say "suffered a stroke"? We don't "suffer" a brain tumor, appendicitis, or gall stones.) Joan visited her friend as soon as she came home from the hospital. June was sitting at the kitchen table rolling out piecrusts with her left hand; her right side is completely paralyzed. The next time Joan came to see her, June was tangled in reams of paper and ribbons, determined to wrap Christmas presents with one hand.

"I wonder if others who have had strokes know what can be done if you try?" thought Joan. She called the Heart Association to see if they knew of support groups in the area and was told that they hadn't much experience with any but would be glad to help if she got one started. She was encouraged to "do her own thing." And with the cooperation and enthusiastic help of her friend, Gail Rapoza, she did. Now, after eight years, people come from all over the greater Hartford area to be a part of this congenial, reassuring group.

As we come into the room, Josephine O'Connor is playing the piano and some have gathered around her. Henry Beaulieu is singing his heart out: "and when Irish eyes are smiling, sure they steal your heart away." The bells ring for me and my gal, the harvest moon shines on, we call everyone sweetheart, and we keep on smiling 'cause when you're smiling, the whole world smiles with you. Then Jo begins the "modern" songs, *our* songs, and with memories in our eyes, we hum along with "I'll be loving you, always," "I'll string along with you," "I'm confessin' that I love you," and "I'll be seeing you in all the old familiar places." Each occasion is a happy, social time with refreshments purchased from a memorial fund given by a former member's family.

Of those who attend a typical meeting, five men and one woman are able to come on their own, two male caregivers bring their wives, and ten men who have had strokes come with their caregivers: wives, sisters, or daughters.

One of the most faithful of the caregiving husbands is Henry Beaulieu. Henry and his wife, Bernadette, of French-Canadian back-ground, both worked at the aircraft factory in East Hartford. Henry was an expediter; Bernadette worked in the Inspection Department. One afternoon when they were visiting us, Henry described the terrible despair he felt the day Berna-

The Phenomenon of Support Groups

dette collapsed at the supermarket and was taken to the hospital.

"When that policeman came to the door and told me where she was, I was numb. I don't know how I got the strength to drive to the hospital but I did. From that day on, I was with her every minute I could be. I would hold her hand and ask her to move her eyelids if she knew me. After forty years of communicating—we never had children so we were everything to each other—after forty years, to get no response—it was awful. When she finally did begin to squeeze my hand and move her eyes, that was stupendous! At night, when I was home alone, I would think 'What's going to happen to us? What kind of future can we have? What is it going to be like for Bernadette? For me?'"

During the direst days, Henry read every book he could find on strokes. Very soon, however, he found out that, in addition to his new medical knowledge, he had to be very practical: he had to find out what kind of soap to use in the dishwasher.

"She never let me come in the kitchen," he laughed. "I didn't even know where the dishwasher *was*. I thought it must be somewhere near the sink. The first time I used it I got the wrong box of stuff and the thing filled the whole room with soap bubbles! What a mess!" He shook his head in disbelief as he remembered his first confrontation with domestic calamity.

After three months, Bernadette was moved to a rehabilitation hospital about thirty-five miles away. "Then I really had my work cut out for me," exclaimed Henry. As he described the days that followed, I relived some of my experiences when Ted was at Jefferson House and felt again the conflict between gratitude for what was being done and the impatience with what I thought were omissions in the kind of care he was getting.

"If her therapy appointment was for nine in the morning, I was there at eight-thirty," Henry explained. "If she wasn't dressed yet, and she usually wasn't, I dressed her and took her down to the therapy room. If the therapist wasn't there by five after nine, I went to talk to the management. I really got angry. Every day they began the treatment late and quit early. Someone was paying for forty-five minutes worth, and we were getting only thirty minutes at the most.

"And another thing"—Henry spoke with deep feeling as he recounted his next clash with the staff—"They sent a psychologist in one day to talk with Bernadette. Bernadette was asleep the whole time. At the end of an hour of the woman talking to me, I asked her if she was being paid to talk to Bernadette. She said yes. I said well, we don't need you. I think that's medical robbery. One afternoon she saw me sitting on the lawn with Bernadette, and she talked to us for a few minutes. She charged for that, too. I complained. I'm a Gemini—I challenge! I figure I'm the caregiver who has to represent the patient who can't represent herself—the patient, and all those guys out there who are paying for what they don't get or don't want. I was there to see that Bernadette got the best care and the best treatment available. I was willing to do the impossible for her—they should be able to do the possible. And I think it paid off. They thought she wouldn't ever walk by herself. Look at how she walked in here today! I pave the way ahead for her, and I follow up behind her in every situation. I back her up, all the way."

"Don't you ever have *any* time off?" I asked.

"When I get a haircut or shop for groceries."

Thinking of all the things I have to do around the house, I asked Henry how he scheduled their days and whether he did all the cooking.

"Oh, sure. I do it because I have to. I found out that kitchen work is no big deal. I'm good at reading recipes and following directions. I must say I threw away a lot of soup at the beginning because I put in too much flour for thickening, but it's okay now. I made some real good onion soup last night. Anyway, in the morning, after I help get Bernadette dressed, I lay out her medication and get her breakfast. She likes French toast a lot. Then we read the paper, check the stock market reports, maybe watch Donahue, snooze a bit, then I help her bathe. After that we take a walk. I carry along a folding chair and every once in awhile we stop so she can rest. After lunch we nap and then usually take a ride someplace. I like to see that she gets out of the house. After dinner in the evening we watch the news. She goes to bed about eight and I watch TV or read or listen to the radio. I go for Pavarotti and Domingo, and symphonies."

"When you travel, what do you do about taking Bernadette to the restroom?" I asked, remembering my hesitant encounters with men's rooms.

"If it's in a restaurant, I usually tell the manager and he sends a waitress in with her. I always tell Bernadette to make sure the floor is not wet in the cubicle, so she won't slip or get her slacks wet when she sits down. And I always tell her to be sure there is toilet paper on the roll before she goes in. I don't want her to get caught in there by herself."

"Henry, you think of more details than anyone I know," I said with admiration. I glanced at Bernadette, who was smiling and nodding in agreement.

"Well," said Henry, "keeping up with the details keeps your mind off the big changes—and there are some big ones. One of the biggest is the change in Bernadette's personality. It used to be when she walked into a room it was like lightning: everybody came around her and she was the spark for the whole bunch. They used to kid her about her claim to fame: her name is on the moon!"

"How's that?" I asked incredulously. I had the same awful fear I had one time with Ted: was someone fantasizing?

"That's the truth," Henry interrupted my thoughts. "As the parts for the lunar landing module were accepted and marked at Pratt and Whitney, her initials were required—she was the records keeper. And there they are—way up there in the sky! B.B."

Henry continued to tell us about Bernadette. "Now she's an introvert, very quiet, not spontaneous the way she used to be. But I promised to care for her in sickness and in health, and that vow means more to me than anything. Oh, sure, I get tired out, emotionally and physically. And there are some really bad times along the way. I used to cry a lot, but I said to myself, 'Henry, no emotion, no devotion.' It's a big job, or course. I tell you, the caregiver has to think a lot about his patient, but he has to think about himself all the time, too."

He looked out of the window at the snow beginning to fall.

"We've got to start home. I cannot be in an accident. I worry about keeping my car in good shape so it would be ready in an emergency. I worry about other drivers on the road, the careless ones. It is just not possible for me to be hurt or sick, and I haven't been—not one day. I just hope God gives me one day more than she gets." I realized then that the greatest thing you can do for someone you love is to outlive them.

As they walked toward the door, Henry smiled. "I used to be just about next to being an atheist. I believed in reality more than spirituality, I guess you'd say. That

The Phenomenon of Support Groups

was four years ago. Now I believe in spirituality more than reality."

As he held Bernadette's arm, directing the use of her quad-cane, and helped her down the steps and into the car, I thought, "Henry, you do a pretty good job of combining both!"

At the Christmas meeting of the Stroke Club, Henry sang "The Lord's Prayer" and "O Holy Night." He has a fine voice. On the table was a beautiful fruitcake he had made for the potluck supper.

In that group, support from each other—those worse off than you, those better off than you—is almost tangible. One learns that surviving takes almost total time, and that a sense of humor and a minimum amount of self-pity are great advantages along the way. In fact, those two attributes almost guarantee the ability to "make it" on the part of both the one who has had the stroke and the one who does the caregiving.

"Ever since I got off the pity-pot, I've made a lot of progress," boasted one man as he moved toward the table in his walker and reached for a piece of Henry's fruitcake.

* * *

"How about coming with me to New Haven this afternoon to a garden party?" I asked a neighbor who has often joined me in spontaneous adventures.

"Of course," she replied.

On an overcast but warm afternoon we set off in the VW convertible with the top down and arrived a bit disheveled in front of a handsome house in a beautifully landscaped yard just north of the Yale campus. I had Jean rehearse carefully the initials of the group giving the party, VSRP, an acronym that is easily confused. For weeks after I had heard it, I stumbled when saying it, but once we were its beneficiaries, it slid easily into our vocabulary.

I had read about the Volunteer Stroke Rehabilitation Program in our newspaper and called the Greater Hartford program director, Peg Laakso, to see if we could fit into it in some way. Shortly after my talk with her, she visited us with Nancy Joyce, a volunteer who lives in Newington and who offered to come once a week to talk with Ted and see if such visits could encourage him to speak more clearly.

The guest of honor at the garden party was the actress Patricia Neal. The book *Pat and Roald,* which describes her rehabilitation after a severe stroke, had been given to me while Ted was in the hospital. Jean and I were introduced to her shortly after we arrived and found her, beautiful and radiant in a bright purple suit, surrounded by stroke survivors and their volunteer companions. She had been the inspiration for VSRP for she exemplified the kind of hope and encouragement that had led Norma Horwitch, founder of the New Haven organization, to realize what help could come for stroke survivors with aphasia.

Aphasia—"loss or impairment of the power to use or understand speech"—occurs frequently when certain areas of the brain are damaged. When Patricia Neal had her stroke several years ago, she emerged with severe aphasia, and only with constant work and the help of many volunteers was her speech returned to normal. Out of these efforts, the British Volunteer Stroke Scheme was organized to give others the kind of aid she had received. Norma Horwitch, a speech therapist, learned of that group and became interested in starting one in the Greater New Haven area. Recognizing the feeling of solitary confinement that traps most aphasic sufferers, she began to organize a community of volunteers who, without formal training, could visit and talk with aphasics regularly and who would have the compassion and willingness to help a person whose "computer brain," as Norma describes it, has temporarily "gone down."

At the party, Jean and I spoke with Patricia Neal briefly, long enough to be impressed with the unique, resonant voice that has brought her accolades in the theater and many film successes. We could see what strides she had made since the time she could not speak a word. The volunteers who pressed around her were inspired also, and were determined to renew their efforts with their particular stroke friends.

"Isn't it wonderful to see what support we have developed in only five years!" exclaimed Norma, looking around the crowded garden. She told me about chapters in New Haven, Waterbury, and Hartford, and of the growing interest in Fairfield County and New York City. "It takes a lot of work to start a VSRP chapter, to find committed people to serve on boards, to hire program coordinators. We have a party like this once or twice a year to get funds for our own group."

Looking around at the enthusiastic faces and pausing for a moment to take in the cheerful chatter arising from the group, Norma mused. "You know—boredom—boredom is one of the evils of stroke. The more stimulating things that can happen day by day, the better a stroke survivor will be in morale and performance. Sometimes our volunteers find that after a few weeks of playing cards or doing puzzles with their companions, the words begin to come. They come so much more naturally when we are all relaxed. Just look," she spread her arms expansively, "look and listen. What a great way to spend an afternoon!"

On the way home I told Jean what Nancy Joyce's visits have meant to Ted. Though he is not aphasic according to the definition, Ted's vocal cords were affected by his stroke so that his speech is slower than before and, unless he concentrates completely, is not always distinct. When Nancy asks him questions, he answers at length and she seems able to understand him better than anyone else, including me. I often think that Nancy knows Ted better than I do for she listens for one solid hour each week as he recounts his activities, tells stories from his childhood, or replies to her questions about history. In my schedule of errands, housekeeping, cooking, shopping, and trying to find time for reading, writing, and walking, I never take a whole hour with Ted to encourage him to talk. When I do ask questions, they tend to be "Did you have a b.m. today?" or "Are you on the last section of the newspaper yet?" so I can prepare his instant cereal.

"What is that book on your table?" asked Nancy at the end of a visit one day.

"That's the yearbook from my senior year in high school," Ted replied.

After we had seen the Winslow Homer watercolors at the Yale Art Gallery, he had pulled it out to show me the "theme" for the 1927 yearbook from West High School, Green Bay, Wis. Each section was introduced by a tableau of students enacting a Winslow Homer painting.

"I'd like for you to show that to me next week," said Nancy, eagerly.

I knew immediately how much that would mean to Ted and wondered why I hadn't thought of it, or rather hadn't taken the time to do it.

Nancy's thoughtfulness and her generosity have been incredibly good therapy for Ted, but more than that, he has found a friend who, for one hour each week, has concentrated on him, his interests, his day, his life.

We who are his family have contributed in other ways, but this special kind of focus is what VSRP has contributed to us and to many others.

Thank you, Patricia Neal, thank you, Norma Horwitch, and thank you, Peg Laakso. But most of all thank you, Nancy Joyce.

CHAPTER IX

Adult Day Care

One Saturday morning as we sat at the breakfast table, Ted said suddenly, out of the blue, "I won a tea bag squeezer."

Completely bewildered, I said, "You *what*?"

"I won a tea bag squeezer at the Halloween party."

I dropped my eyes and tried to collect myself. Was he beginning to be incoherent? Was he hallucinating? Had the day I dreaded most of all arrived? "Was it a dream, Ted? What was the rest of the dream? Tell me about the party in that dream."

"No, it wasn't a dream," he said, a bit impatiently. "I won the tea bag squeezer at our Halloween party at the day care center yesterday. I won it because I knew the name of the song Tina played—it was 'Till We Meet Again.'"

I jumped up from the table.

"Good for you!" I shouted, in an entirely new context. I think he was understandably perplexed at the intensity of the hug I gave him, just for recognizing "Till We Meet Again."

His prize had been won at the Betty Larus Adult Day Care Center in Hartford, about two miles from our home, where he goes one day a week. He agrees to this break in his daily routine for my sake for he knows how much the one free day means to me. Always, if given a choice, he says he would prefer to stay at home, but he has now accepted the fact that his day away gives me a few uninterrupted hours when I can write, read, or squander rare, unscheduled time. We pay $33.00 a day for him to be there, which includes a full dinner at noon. He goes at nine and I usually pick him up about four in the afternoon.

It was very hard at first when I had to balance my great desire for time for myself against Ted's reluctance to spend the day away from his books and comfortable room. In those early days, when I would come for him, I would find him sitting alone, just waiting, waiting for me to come, and I would feel very guilty, making him endure this. Since that time, I have learned that he spends quite a busy day at the center, and among other activities, he has found someone who will play Scrabble with him after the day's formal program is over. Sometimes I have to wait quite a while for him to finish a close game.

"Marge beat me by two points today, but I think she practices at home. She's good!" he said one day.

I remember when a friend first suggested that Ted could attend an adult day care center, I thought we had come full circle: a nursery school-type setup with games, music, and snacks at the end of life as at the beginning. But when I found out more about this recent phenomenon—day care for the chronically ill or disabled, for those who are convalescing, or for those living alone without many social contacts—I realized it is on a very different level from any nursery school. The variety of activities, opportunities for mental stimulation and social interaction, the valuable health services provided regularly—these are of immeasurable help to the participants who contribute to the group from diverse backgrounds and experience. Equally valuable is the chance for caregivers to have time off from their responsibilities and be free from anxiety about the care their "patient" is being given. Needless to say, I am an enthusiastic advocate for this relatively new institution in our society.

I was surprised to find out that the center Ted attends—the first one in Connecticut—was organized as recently as 1971. Now there are more than forty. The staff includes a registered nurse, a social worker, a therapeutic recreation director, aides, and bus drivers, all supervised by a creative, dynamic administrator, Beth Hugh.

"Do you realize," she asked me one day when I was talking to her about the makeup of this special community, "that those who are over 85 are the fastest-growing age group in our population? Can you imagine how many more two-career families there will be who are going to find themselves with an aging parent in their homes? Or how many ninety-year-olds with broken hips there will be, not to mention the almost insolvable home problems that will arise from the increasing number of Alzheimer's patients?"

I was overwhelmed by the prospects and determined to find out more about the program Beth Hugh directs.

"Tell me what you do during the day at the center," I asked Ted one day.

"First we do exercises with Kitty—ones I can do in my wheelchair. Then we have toast and coffee in the dining room. The movies come next [Ted chooses to attend on Fridays because on that day they have movies, mostly documentaries]. Today they had one on Copenhagen—I was the only one who had been there—and another had clips of old movies. One of them had Ruth Roland in it."

Adult Day Care

"Ruth who?"

"Ruth Roland. I used to see her movies when I was a kid in Milwaukee." I listened carefully for he doesn't often reminisce.

"My mother used to take in roomers, and there was this cabinetmaker who lived on the third floor." I leaned toward him to be sure I didn't miss any part of the story. "He used to pay me 5¢ a week to bring him the *Milwaukee Leader*—it was a Socialist newspaper. With that money I'd go to the Saturday matinee and watch Ruth Roland. I saw her then for 5¢; today I saw her for $33.00."

"Let's get back to the program at day care. What did you have for lunch?"

"Seafood newburg, broccoli, rice, apple pie, and coffee."

"No salad?" I asked.

"I wouldn't eat salad even if they had it. You know that," he retorted.

"With whom did you sit at the table?"

"I don't know their names." I made a mental note to suggest introductions or name tags.

"What about the afternoon?"

"We have exercises with Lena, upstairs. After that, before I play Scrabble with Marge, we have a snack."

"What were those women doing at the table when I came to get you?"

"Making posters for the fair next Saturday. I forgot—this afternoon they took our blood pressure. Mine was 123 over 61. And when they weighed us, I found out I'd gained two pounds since last time." I thought I detected a bit of pride in his voice.

"Good for you," I exclaimed. "What about that notice on the bulletin board about a trip to the museum. Can you do that?"

"Yes. They have a van that takes the wheelchairs. And the week after that trip we're going to visit another day care center in West Hartford, where they are having a musical program."

Ted was among a few from his day care group who were chosen to take part in a series of classes conducted by the Connecticut Department on Aging on the subject "Family Album: the American Family in Literature and History." One day, after their session on "Death and Dying," I asked Ted how the class went: had he contributed to the discussion?

"Well, I'm an old John Dewey man," he explained. "I believe in learning by doing."

That ended *that*.

Though at first Ted had accepted the day care days reluctantly, I could see that he was beginning to look forward to his Fridays, the now not-so-unwelcome interruption in his reading routines, a sociability with new people in an environment I do not share, and an independence from which we are both benefiting.

As we arrived one morning, Liz, the staff social worker, was getting out of her car with a bulging plastic bag in one hand.

"Guess what's happened to us," she said enthusiastically. "We've been awarded the Pom Pom franchise for the Dog Grooming Salon!"

"What kind of franchise?" I asked.

"This friend of mine runs a dog-grooming place and will pay us to make the yarn pom-poms they attach to the dogs' collars when they finish grooming them. We get 50¢ a pom-pom and have to make 150 every two weeks. We'll use the profits to take more trips."

Sure enough, when I came to get Ted that afternoon, most of the women and two of the men were sitting at a table winding yarn around two discs, cutting it, and fluffing it into varicolored puffs.

"The little ones are for poodles," explained Mary Esther, a small, stoop-shouldered lady whom I had met earlier, "and the big ones are for the big dogs. And the color is supposed to match the dog," she said, emphatically.

The busy craftspeople did not seem to disturb Ted and Marge's Scrabble game. Ted was wearing his "I Don't Do Crafts" button, a treasured gift from a sympathetic friend.

One day after we'd returned from a vacation, I was shopping at the supermarket when a woman I had seen at the center came running up to me.

"Tell Ted Marilyn is all right now. She had her operation last week and is getting along fine."

I reported this conversation to Ted with a little hesitation and some concern. Though I don't know the names of all his friends at the center, I assumed Marilyn was one of his Friday companions. I was puzzled, therefore, to see his face break out in a big grin.

"Marilyn is the black cat that came to the center one day, and we just adopted her," he explained matter-of-factly.

I began to want to know more about the people who need adult day care. I knew that the personnel committee at the center wants to get a diversified case mix, as well as to provide both a comfortable place where those who are forgetful or confused can spend the day and a supervised situation where the physically disabled but mentally alert can find needed assistance and sociability.

"I come five days a week," Ernie told me when I asked him what he likes about day care. "I was paralyzed after my stroke in February. Now I can get around in this wheelchair. I'm only sixty-one so I wasn't retired yet. If I stayed at home all day I would drive my nieces crazy. Here I can get a bath once a week; they have that whirlpool I can get into."

I recognized one woman as the mother of a boy who had gone to grade school with our daughter, Marcia. "I heard about this place when I was doing volunteer work," said Ciel when I visited with her. "Then, when I had my stroke—well, come to think of it I've had two strokes—my husband works every day and even though my daughter moved in with us to help take care of me, she works every day, so what would I do if I couldn't come here? I don't have any paralysis, so I can get around all right, but my memory is sort of dull. They don't want me to be alone all day. This is a good place to be."

One morning when I took Ted, I met Michael, a retired university teacher who has Parkinson's disease. He is working on a special project: he is writing his autobiography—a long, slow process. And for a few weeks, a young thirty-three-year-old social worker who was recovering from an aneurysm in her brain came to the center until she was well enough to return to work.

"This has been my home for seven years now," said Mary Esther, looking up from the tablecloth she was embroidering. "I live alone in the housing for the elderly in Hartford; we have a regular League of Nations there. The van picks me up on Monday, Wednesday, and Friday."

Just then Marilyn came over and jumped in her lap. "She likes me a lot," Mary Esther smiled. "Now don't get tangled up in my thread," she warned. And to me, "I like to embroider. I do a lot of cross-stitch." Then she winked. "I don't knit, only when the doctor cuts me up. I've had a lot of doctors but most of them are dead now. I was born in convulsions, had infantile paralysis when I was a baby. When I was older I had a compound fracture when I was hit by a drunken driver. A few years after that I had a hysterectomy—I think that's what you call it—and you can see by this big bump on my back that I have scoliosis. How many times I've heard them say 'we almost lost you,' but here I am today! The van brings me here for day care, but other times I have to call Dial-a-Ride to go to the doctor or to Bingo. That's funny, isn't it? They'll take me to Bingo in Dial-a-Ride but not to my hairdresser. I have to take a cab for that. You know," she called as I stood to leave, "I don't drink or drive. I do say 'damn' once in a while."

The van then arrived to take Mary Esther back to her one room in the Tower for the Elderly and to take Alice, completely disoriented—her only words all day are "Merry Christmas, Virginia"—back to the home where she lives with her son and daughter-in-law, a banker and an insurance officer. Ernie's niece was just driving up to take him to his newly ramped house. I urged Ted and Marge to decide who was having the last word so I could take Ted home to his Talking Book and his evening newspaper.

Once, when we were talking about problems of the aging at a Quaker conference, one of our friends said, "I wish you could see our adult day care center. I volunteer there once a week, and it is the best thing I've done since we retired. Come in the fall and meet some of the folks who make this such a special place."

We explained that Ted was part of such a center in Hartford, that it means a great deal to us, and that we would very much like to see another center.

On a golden October day we drove about forty miles southwest of Hartford to Southbury to see what River

Glen Adult Day Care, part of the River Glen Continuing Care Center, offers its participants. Patricia Rockwell, the director, was eager to share her enthusiasm for her job. As I sat in her office I could see our friend Millie challenge the group of people who sat in a semicircle around the blackboard.

"All right, now," said Millie brightly. "We're doing fruits and vegetables. What vegetable can you get out of l-e-g-n-a-t-g-p?" That took a few minutes, but the next one, "a-e-f-g-p-r-t-r-i-u" was guessed almost immediately. When they began a game with history question, Ted was the star student.

"Eighty percent of our people have Alzheimer's, 18 percent have had strokes, and others have miscellaneous disabilities," said Patricia. "Because there are different levels of Alzheimer's, we try to have games as mentally stimulating as possible to be sure those who *are* able can keep their minds working. Here is one of our most successful games: 'Ungame.'" She handed me a small white card with a question on it: "If you had to move and could take only three things with you, what would you take?"

"We got some interesting answers on that one," Patricia smiled.

"Now this one really brings out a lot of emotional response. We learn a great deal about each other when we draw this card: 'When was the last time you cried and why?'"

After the games were finished and some people were being wheeled toward the bathrooms before lunch, I asked about the music we were hearing in the background and to which some in the room were listening attentively.

"The husband of one of our long-time participants

Adult Day Care

wanted to do something for the center after his wife died, so he gave us a complete set of eighteen cassettes: 'Music Masters—in Story and Music.' Each tape tells stories about the composer and then intersperses them with his music. We got these tapes from a children's catalog. You'd be surprised how many fascinating things there are in 'Toys to Grow On' for our purposes."

I asked if there were other ways in which families were involved in their program.

"We have started two support groups. One is for families and friends of our Alzheimer patients. We have a sitter service for them so families can be free to come to the meetings. Those people gain immense strength from each other for, as you know, that disease is one of the most grueling for the caregivers."

"And the second support group?" I asked.

"You might not think we need this one, but it has been a great help. We have an adult day care support group for the families of people who come here in order to explain our program and help them understand some of the things we do. Many times they get an inaccurate picture of what goes on here. And, of course, it helps us to know the people who are caring for those we see here day after day."

As we rose to go to lunch, Patricia said a little wistfully, "We have a hard row to hoe between those who are getting better and are able to do more things week after week, and those whose decline becomes more obvious, almost from day to day."

Lunch was in a very sunny, pleasant dining room (it is surprising what a difference a cloth tablecloth makes!). We sat at a table with a medical librarian who was paralyzed after a fall from a balcony when he was traveling in Italy. He puts his electric scooter in his car and ships both to Florida with him for the winter. There he is able to get around very easily. "Fewer hills," he explains, "and *everything* is ramped. Here, on these Connecticut slopes, it's a little risky."

As we drove back to Hartford on a back road lined with gold, yellow, and green trees, Ted and I talked of the privileged people whom we had met that day. All at River Glen at this time are private patients paying twenty-six dollars a day. We worried together about the hundreds of elderly who need therapeutic care as well as the socialization of a warm community group, and about their caregivers, who need a few hours release from their daily obligation. We wondered where the funds were coming from to pay for the solutions to these needs.

CHAPTER X

Problems: Financial and Otherwise

I was shocked, as many are, to discover what Medicare does not cover: there are no provisions for adult day care, and there are very limiting restrictions on remuneration for nursing home care. Increasing numbers of people who are above the poverty level are forced to "spend down"— to exhaust their own resources to pay the costs of long-term nursing home care or of home care for those who are valiantly trying to stay in their own homes as long as they possibly can. They watch the savings they have accumulated during a lifetime for their "golden" retirement years disappear in no time at all. I remembered the panicky feeling I had when Ted was at Jefferson House, realizing it would take our entire annual income to keep him there each year.

In the day care center Ted attends, 35 percent of the group are on Medicaid, which means that all their savings have been used up and they are eligible for welfare. Others must pay from their own resources, knowing how much less these expenses are than the $80-$120 a day one must pay in a convalescent or nursing home.

Is there no one in our society who is paying attention to these problems? Are those in charge of making decisions and creating new programs all too young to have experienced the terrors of a parent with Alzheimer's or the helpless look on the face of a paralyzed friend? Just as I was asking myself these questions, a story appeared in the paper describing new responses by some who *are* concerned.

One new concept would require employees and possibly employers to put dollars in an account during their working years, and on retirement, the accumulated funds plus interest would finance health care for life, including home health care. A proposal by the secretary of health and human services suggested an annual contribution of $1,000, for example, by a young couple. It sounded good until I added up the figures and discovered that, if one saved that amount for thirty-five years it would cover only a portion of the time a person would need to be in a nursing home. I also remembered our state of mind at age thirty. Buying a home, paying on a car, planning for the children's education—it would have been impossible for us to have liberated $1,000 a year for those far-off expenses of a nursing home. We wouldn't have had those extra funds, and besides, at *that* time, we could never imagine ourselves being old and needing anything *like* a nursing home!

When I called the state insurance commissioner's office to find out what the situation is in our state, I was told that perhaps soon there will be some kind of insurance program marketed for continuing care coverage for the elderly, but as of now only a few states have such policies, and provisions for custodial care are almost nonexistent. The premiums he quoted as examples of what might be required were astoundingly high.

Are there other plans? I discovered that at Brandeis University, the Heller School has been awarded a grant to develop a prepaid system of care for the elderly that has come to be known as a social/health maintenance organization (S/HMO, pronounced *schmoe*).*

These plans are for the elderly, of course, those eligible for Medicare or Medicaid. But somehow strokes and other disabilities don't limit themselves to those over sixty-five. Where are funds going to come from for those who are not fortunate enough to live in states where insurance companies are allowed to offer policies that help cover continuing care costs and who do not qualify for government programs?

What about the sandwich generation—those with children to finance on the one hand and elderly parents on the other, with increasing college costs coming at a time when there are increasing health care costs? What about Ted and me, should he need to be in a nursing home again—a prospect we couldn't possibly afford? What about the surprising information given me recently by the day care administrator: the two main reasons a person is admitted to a nursing home are that either he or she becomes incontinent or, and this is the frightening prospect, the caregiver gives out!

Respite care—adult day care centers, short-term arrangements in convalescent or nursing homes, live-in help during brief vacation breaks—should be high in the priorities of any continuing care policies. Who is considering the vast amounts that could be saved, both privately and publicly, for a small investment in the kind of care that could diminish the stress that often accompanies the caregiver's role and that can lead to such costly results?

*Several places in the country—e.g., Brooklyn, N.Y.; Portland, Oreg.; Minneapolis, Minn.; Long Beach, Calif.—are sponsoring demonstration sites where a single provider organization assumes responsibility for a full range of services.

I spent one snowy November morning talking with Lucy Townsend, the very bright, efficient director of a promising pioneer program called Connecticut Community Care, Inc., a private nonprofit organization that provides case management to elderly persons and disabled children and adults. A corps of nurses and social workers evaluates their clients, recommends creative options that will encourage independent living as often as possible, and monitors their services. These include visiting nurses, therapists, part-time help from volunteers, or, in some instances, adult day care. Financial resources to be explored and tapped include church funds, charitable trusts, veterans groups, and community agencies. There is a sliding scale of fees for those not eligible for Medicaid or assistance from state agencies for the aging. I saw this kind of program as a helpful resource, albeit an expensive one, for those of us not quite needy enough for state aid.

This is a long way from Ted's tea bag squeezer and his memory of Saturday matinees with Ruth Roland. We are so lucky to have our Fridays. Without this one uninterrupted day of the week, I could not have written an article—or this book. But what of all the others who need relief from their twenty-four-hour duties?

If we can find millions of dollars to send to victims of floods or earthquakes in an emergency, we surely have the resources and the imagination to figure out ways to finance care for those who need it. Who knows, it may take on the proportions of a national disaster if we do not plan ahead with compassion and concern now.

* * *

"Who cares for the caregiver?" is asked more and more often these days by the community of social workers who

Problems: Financial and Otherwise

have added this title to their vocabulary (more friendly sounding than *caretaker*) and by those of us—husbands, wives, sisters, brothers, nurses, doctors, neighbors, and friends—who find ourselves in this category.

We are well aware of the stresses to which we are subject, the added responsibilities we have to accept, the daily and nightly demands that have interrupted our agendas, the unplanned emergencies, and the painful decision making. Some of us have been recently made aware, in articles and speeches, of the fact that those who wish to help us may sometimes be deterred by a kind of shield of invulnerability with which we surround ourselves. The strength we think we must have to be able to "do it all" may intimidate some who have not yet been called upon to exhibit that kind of desperate determination. Those of us engaged in "continuing care" have to beware of the dangers of a kind of "spiritual arrogance" which, unintentionally, tends to set us apart when we most need encouragement and reinforcement. We need to seek support in groups that offer it, to accept kindnesses gratefully, to learn to say "no" or "yes" with grace. In addition, we must learn that protecting our own physical and emotional health is a responsibility we ignore at our peril. When we come right down to the final answer to the question above, the person who cares for the caregiver is the caregiver.

Our physical health is a priority, of course, and when we are rational and clearheaded we know in the back of our minds that good food, enough sleep, time for "rest and relaxation," alone-time, and help with tedious duties all contribute to our well-being. But finding ways to implement these requirements is not always so easy.

I've looked for practical helps along the way, which have made the onerous tasks lighter, and I have *tried* to incorporate regular exercise into a busy schedule. For instance, when I found that lifting Ted's wheelchair into the back of the car was getting to be too much of a burden, we were able to get a lightweight titanium one with features that make it easy to fit into any kind of vehicle. We considered a motorized scooter such as Hugh Johnson uses with such pleasure, but it was much too heavy for me to maneuver into the car if we wanted to take it with us, and its use in town was limited to places where there are ramped sidewalks and entryways.

As for exercise, I found that a new twelve-speed bike was a wonderful way to ride to the library, much more tempting than my forty-year-old three-speed, which was a real whiz in its day. As for walking, I discovered that listening to books-on-tape on my Walkman as I took my outings meant that I became so interested in *Passage to India* or *Proof* or *School for Scandal* that I walked miles farther. A swimnastics class or cross-country skiing when possible offer a different kind of reward for body and soul. My devotion to Zone Therapy (massaging my ears, hands, and feet before I get out of bed in the morning) makes a real difference in the way I greet the day. And Jane Fonda's Low Impact Aerobic Workout has me "washing windows" and doing the hula in the living room in any weather that's not clement.

All this exercise—even the thought of it—is anathema to Ted, who has always been a devotee of Robert Hutchins's philosophy: when he feels the need to exercise coming over him, he lies down until it passes away. Getting Ted onto the exercycle or suggesting that he follow the Wheelchair Workout (see bibliography) gives me a lot of exercise—in persuasion. I once observed that the only workout he practices consistently and without any urging is shrugging his shoulders, and I'm not sure

Problems: Financial and Otherwise

that is aerobic enough for his ailments these days.

One of the happier innovations in our social life is the practice of buying season tickets to concerts and plays in threes instead of twos, inviting a different person to accompany us for each performance. What a joy it is to have someone along to open a door, help lift the wheelchair into the station wagon, wait with Ted while I park the car, and take an arm so we can walk into a restaurant without the wheelchair. And postmortems of shows are always more interesting when a third voice joins in. Of course, we do things in fours also, but often a single person is freer to fit into our schedule.

There are many practical material things, both large and small, that the caregiver gives thanks for daily. For me, a built-in laundry comes first: I am still in awe of those miraculous inventions, a washer and a dryer. I remember the years I helped my mother run the clothes through the wringer from the washer to the rinse water (I once included my arm with the sheets), through the wringer from the rinse water to the bluing water, through the wringer from the bluing water to the huge clothes basket, which we then carried to the clothesline in the backyard. I don't know what I would have done these last few years if I had to go through those processes with the mountains of sheets, towels, and clothes I've had to wash.

High on the gratitude list are electric-eye doors that open on approach—what a difference they make for a wheelchair user. Yet as valuable as that electronic gadget is, even more so is the eye of the thoughtful bystander who, without a word, runs to open the door in front of us. How we bless that person!

There are lots of insignificant things that become significant: zip-lock bags in which to store leftovers; door braces that hold screen and storm doors open; *instant* anything: cereal, coffee, soup, boiling water, cocoa, pudding, protein supplement. And always the best of friends, Ensure, the meal-in-a-can, which means that Ted can get his own meal if I need to be gone.

These are some of the practical helps for both of us, aids to our physical and mental health. Our emotional health is nurtured by a constant outflowing of love and concern, by friends who reach out in so many ways to encourage and help us. Particularly appreciated are the notes that end, "you don't need to acknowledge this" (such understanding usually inspires a desire to answer immediately), and the oh-so-welcome-if-brief frequent phone calls "just checking in." They mean so much; it is hard to imagine how gratitude for them can be adequately expressed.

Providing a stimulating environment is another facet of emotional health and one that is often a real challenge for the caregiver. The great temptation that we often have, and that Ted would gladly follow, is the path of least resistance. It is one of my more difficult chores to find that fine line between variety and rest, to balance the days between social commitments and time that would otherwise be devoid of contacts with others.

One morning when I outlined the day's schedule, Ted reacted with intense feeling. "Horrors, horrors. O horrors!" At noon we were to attend the luncheon for emeritus professors at the college. In the late afternoon we were to visit one of the historians Ted had hired, who was retiring and moving to Florida. That evening we had tickets for *A Doll's House* at the Hartford Stage Company. An additional feature for the day was the weather: icy rain made sidewalks and driveways sheets of sleet. It would have been easy to stay home from one or all of the

Problems: Financial and Otherwise

above, but we didn't, and after the luncheon Ted said, "I was glad to hear about those new buildings the president talked about." After our visit with Michael and Helena: "That was such a good time. I'll miss them." And after the play: "That was good. That Nora was very different from the other Noras I've seen. I liked that."

Of course, we were both tired that night, but it had not been *so* horrible, all those activities, and there was no schedule at all for the next day. We would have a whole twenty-four hours to rest up for all the things we planned to do the day after that.

CHAPTER XI

Journeying in '86

Exultation is the going
Of an inland soul to sea....
            —Emily Dickinson

Ted had shown great interest in the coming of Halley's comet in 1986, reminding us that Mark Twain had said he had come in with the comet and expected to depart with it, as he did. Ted had come in with it in 1910, the year Mark Twain died, and decided he would like to see it in case he, also, was going to fulfill Mark Twain's prediction.

We decided to take a cruise that combined "comet sighting" in the Caribbean with a trip through the Panama Canal. Our friend, Martha Jean Erb, decided on the same cruise so we developed a "troika," which worked beautifully as there was always an arm to help balance Ted wherever necessary. Both of us helped him get to the top deck where the telescopes were, and one dark night in Aruba we did indeed see a smudge in the night sky, which, the astronomer-on-board assured us, was Halley's comet. Ted's wheelchair barely fit the corridors of the ship, but he could make his way down the halls to the elevators to get to the dining room and upper deck. We were able to take him in the wheelchair when we made shore trips at Cartagena and Acapulco, but he wasn't able to climb down the wobbly ladder to get into the tender to visit the San Blas Islands. That was one place where the trio worked wonderfully, as I spent the morning on the island among the picturesque Cuna Indians, and "M.J." took the afternoon tender after spending the morning with Ted.

In the years since Ted's stroke, he has gained strength so that he can walk short distances with assistance though his balance hasn't improved enough for him to stand or walk alone. Since walking with a walker or cane always necessitates a companion to steady or catch him when he tends to fall to one side, we soon decided it is easier to take his arm and walk with him rather than try to manage cumbersome equipment.

With some trepidation he and I flew one summer to Pine Woods on Higgins Lake in Michigan, our son-in-law's family's summer place. We weren't sure how we were going to negotiate the root-interrupted path through the woods to the dining hall, but we found we could drive from our cottage directly to the back door of the spacious hall, and Ted could manage the buffet line in his wheelchair easily. We also discovered that the pontoon boat, appropriately named "The Geriatica," was a perfect means of lake transportation for someone in a wheelchair. Karen and Phil even persuaded Ted that a canoe trip was possible with lots of helping hands at the beginning and end of the voyage.

When we attended a weekend alumni seminar (available to parents as well as alums) at Karen's alma mater, Middlebury College in Vermont, we were surprised to find that the college had put down great slabs of plywood to facilitate our mobility across the lawns at Breadloaf, the conference center. The morning lecture sessions lasted more than three hours, but if I parked the car near the basement door of the room where Ted was hearing lectures on botany, politics, ballads, and economics, he could get to it during intermission to use his urinal. This enabled me to take in the full morning session on Emily Dickinson, which was clear across the campus.

As we drove home, down Vermont's beautiful Route 100, Ted asked me, hesitantly, "What about Australia?"

"Well, you did so well at Breadloaf," I said, "I'll bet we could do it. I'll talk to Edith this week. We could plan to go next April and see what their autumn is like," I added, looking at the beginning golden tinges on the roadside maples.

So in those September days, our undiscouraged travel agent pulled out our folder and began to make plans for our trip Down Under in the spring. It would be a journey we had looked forward to for a very long time.

* * *

I am constantly thankful, as I was that first night of the stroke, when I assess Ted's deficits. We try to make the many adjustments necessary to accommodate the problems in coordination, but we do not have to make adjustments for any deficits in cognition. An example of a sort of "journey of the mind" occurred in early October.

"Say, I just got an extra copy of my master's thesis from the binders. I'd like for Ted to read it, if he'd be interested." The telephone call was from an energetic, widely traveled insurance executive friend of ours, retired, who had taken a master's degree between his trips as a consultant to Indonesia, Hungary, and many other countries. "The topic of the thesis is 'The Fall Line in American History.'"

Ted read the thesis conscientiously, and one fine autumn day I drove him to Dick's house to discuss it. Dick's wife, Virginia, and I talked in one room while Dick waited eagerly for Ted's appraisal in the living room. We couldn't help but overhear the retired history professor's conclusions:

"You know, Dick, if this thesis were presented to me for a master's, I wouldn't accept it. You have not used any primary sources. You have discussed the Fall Line as a determinant in American history but that is just *your own* assumption. The purpose of a thesis or a dissertation is an exercise in research. It teaches you a technique; it is not supposed to be a soapbox. Frederick Jackson Turner used to come to class with a fist full of notes. He had spent the morning in the library taking them from original sources, and he would just sit there and read from the notes so his students would learn what was available to them."

Dick was a little stunned but took the evaluation in good spirits. After some protestations on his part, a long discussion of the Fall Line by both men, and a rustling of papers, we heard Dick ask, "Anything more, Ted?"

"Yes, Dick, here's the word *unprecedented*: you have misspelled it. And in the last paragraph on page 52, it should be 1717, not 1716."

"Well, I'll bring you more theses to read," said Dick appreciatively. "That would be a good occupation for a wise old historian in a wheelchair, don't you think?"

"If I'd wanted to do that, I wouldn't have retired," snorted Ted.

That same month we traveled to Madison, Wis., for the sixtieth anniversary of the founding of the House Fellows program at the university. Ted had been head fellow at Adams Hall from 1933 to 1935 and was one of the oldest of the alumni who returned for the weekend celebration. After the welcoming party on Friday evening, at which present house fellows performed skits and music, we visited the "Memorabilia Room," which had pictures and news stories of the sixty years of dormitory life at Madison. While I was looking up stories of the thirties in some of the bulging scrapbooks on the center table, I glanced across the room to see Ted surrounded by four students, all presently house fellows in their dorms. A very pretty young woman was kneeling in front of Ted's wheelchair and animatedly talking with him. I stood in the background listening as they plied him with questions, watching their astonishment as they heard his answers.

"You mean you had to wear jackets and ties to dinner every night?"

"Girls had to be in by 10:30?"

"No one could sit down at dinner until the resident fellow sat down?"

They were incredulous.

"But what did you do for *fun*?"

For an hour the students patiently listened to Ted describe a world completely unknown to them. If they didn't understand his words they asked him, without any hesitation, to repeat them. He had to answer their questions about Prohibition, as unbelievable to them as their problems with anorexia, drugs, and drinking were to him.

I was struck with their obviously sincere interest in life in Madison fifty years ago, their persistence in questioning Ted when most people give up after finding they can't understand all his words, their wisdom and understanding in kneeling to his level to talk (something most of us don't think about). I came away that night with complete admiration for the compassion and curiosity of those students, and a keen realization of what it must have meant to Ted to be the object of their attention and to be, for a short time, the authority on dorm life of half a century ago.

The next night we attended the Wisconsin-Michigan football game at Camp Randall, the huge university stadium. On the way, Ted pointed out the tower of the Congregational church rising high above the west side of the stadium, where he had climbed the perilous steps in the belfry to watch football games when he had sold his season ticket to get extra money.

Driving the rented car through the crowd-clogged streets to the stadium took a bit of skill. Talking the policeman into letting us park in the special-permit zone (without our handicapped sticker, which had been left in Connecticut) took even more skill, and pushing the wheelchair up three ramps to the handicapped seating area took just plain strength and will power. We found ourselves with twelve wheelchairs or electric scooters behind a bench on which sat twelve caregivers—two men and ten women. Each occupant had a different disability. Most poignant to me was the handsome young man with a stocking cap pulled low over his forehead against the cold: there were two empty sleeves in his ski jacket. In front of him sat a beautiful young girl who watched the game without changing her expression. At half-time, she went to his side and turned up the stocking cap so he could see without tipping his head. I was overcome by the helpless feeling of having no hands with which to push a cap out of your eyes. At the very end, when Wisconsin made a touchdown and the stadium erupted in a roar, I was deafened by my neighbor—by the sound of no hands clapping. All of us packed our belongings and our blankets into our capacious tote bags and, motorized or hand pushed, worked our way down the ramps, through the crowds, to our cars.

Ted and I enjoyed every minute of that Big Ten game, but it was not always thus. One area in which our interests have diverged is sports. Our travels toward mutual sharing in that field have taken many years! Ted's avid following of baseball and football games had always remained a mystery to me, just as my interests in ice dancing and sailboats have not attracted him. In the year 1986, he watched on television or heard broadcast on the radio 108 Red Sox baseball games. The season was climaxed when Karen took him to Fenway Park in Boston to see his beloved Sox play the second game of the play-offs with the California Angels. I had become involved in the game also, finding I could get a lot of needlework done while watching, and enjoying the companionship. When the celebrating erupted at the end of the World Series, I followed the proceedings to the bitter end—bitter because our team had lost, but still entertaining because of the post-game activities.

"Aren't you going to stay and hear the interviews in the locker room?" I asked as I saw Ted turn to leave the room.

"No," he said, wheeling his wheelchair into the room where the second television is. "I want to see how the Giants are getting along."

And so I followed along into the football season, finally learning the difference between Marino and Montana, erupting in cheers or boos when appropriate, and listening to Ted patiently explain to me why more punts aren't blocked.

Imagine my surprise when I came to the table one morning and Ted announced, "French Kiss beat America II yesterday—they're now in second place, right behind Kiwi Magic." So after the Giants had won the Superbowl, together we began to follow the magnificent telecasts from Australia as Kookaburra III pursued Stars and Stripes and that coveted bulbous silver pitcher, the America's Cup.

When "Tip" O'Neill retired as Speaker of the House of Representatives in Washington, I read one interview in which he described an evening with his wife, Millie: "We sit there and can have a conversation, read and watch the Red Sox. That's what love is all about, especially when you're both in your seventies.

To my great surprise, I have discovered that that, indeed, can be what love is all about.

CHAPTER XII

January '87 Setback

Presentiment–is that long Shadow–on the Lawn–
Indicative that Suns go down–

The Notice to the startled Grass
That Darkness–is about to pass–

—Emily Dickinson

In January 1987, I was standing at the sink, adding boiling water to the instant cereal (I hate to wash cereal pans) and thinking, "This quiet, daily routine has been undisturbed for quite a long time. I wonder how much longer it can go on."

The season of colds and flu was always a season for Ted to be wary: emphysema and bronchiectasis had been his companions for years. In this last month, when he began to cough a lot, I noticed that he was also getting short of breath with each exertion though he showed no signs of a cold. His coughs were mostly unproductive; since the stroke, it has been hard for him to expel mucus from his lungs. When he complained of a queasy stomach on the way to the day care center on January 9, I was concerned enough to pick him up early in the afternoon. On the way home he announced, "My breath is like a young boy."

"How is that?" I asked.

"It comes in short pants."

His labored breathing continued until Monday, and on

that morning I called Dr. Greenglass. "Bring him in at 11:45" was his response.

When the doctor showed us the X rays he had just taken of Ted's lungs, Ted remarked, "In all the years I've had my lungs X-rayed, this is the first time I've ever seen the results." The doctor pointed out the little branches of bronchi, which showed white where they should have been dark, meaning no air was getting through. "The bronchiectasis is pretty widespread," he explained, "and, of course, the emphysema.... Because of Ted's scarred lungs, his X rays are very hard to read." He prescribed a stronger antibiotic.

The medicine did not work miracles, and one night about two weeks later I found Ted gasping for breath. I tried cupping and clapping on his back, and suggested he try to breathe slower and more deeply. Finally his breathing, though labored, was regular enough for him to be able to sleep. I stayed in the living room and checked on him almost hourly.

The next morning I called Dr. Greenglass to see if he thought oxygen might help. He explained that we would have to take him to the pulmonary lab at the hospital for a test of blood gases to determine if he could take oxygen and, if so, how much. The HMO appointments secretary called to say that because of the impending snowstorm, all afternoon appointments had been moved up to the morning and they would be unable to take Ted until the next week. Ted had been so short of breath that morning that he could hardly dress himself. When I wheeled him into the kitchen, he quietly told me that January 22 was going to be his last day on earth. I assured him that it didn't need to be, and with a bit of Henry Beaulieu's spirit waving me on, I called the secretary back and said in a very determined voice that I would go to any lab in any hospital and pay any cost to see if Ted could have oxygen. I realized that when the tough get going, the going gets tough for everyone else!

In fifteen minutes I got a call saying the lab at Hartford Hospital would take us immediately. On that cold, gray, threatening morning, Karen and I got Ted to the lab and home again before the almost-blizzard set in. An hour later Dr. Greenglass called back to say that the test indicated Ted would benefit from oxygen and that it would be delivered that afternoon.

In the height of a swirling snowstorm, the big white truck from the medical supply service arrived, and two attendants brought in a huge tank of oxygen with fifty feet of plastic tubing attached and set it up in Ted's bedroom. I was astounded, for I thought of "oxygen" as a little portable bottle one could carry under one's arm or, at most, a container on wheels such as a friend of ours pulled around with her because of asthma attacks. This system was formidable! Warning signs were posted on the outside of the front and back doors:

> Caution—oxygen in use—no sparks,
> no open flames, no oil or grease—no smoking

We entered the oxygen era!

Ted napped soundly with the little turquoise prongs in his nostrils, and that evening he was able to propel himself, his lap filled with plastic tubing, into the dining room. He quickly resumed his after-dinner reading habit, listened to *Pet Sematary* on Talking Books, and slept well during the night.

When I got to the kitchen the next morning, I found him up, dressed, and ready for the day. I was so relieved that I wept as I hugged him. What a difference to see him breathing well and responding to the beautiful snow-

January '87 Setback

covered world with his old spirit. "But I couldn't have gotten dressed without this," he said, lifting the tube. "I tried taking it off and couldn't get breath enough to put my clothes on."

Saturday morning, as requested by Dr. Greenglass, a nurse came from the Visiting Nurse and Home Care Association. She explained the benefits of the right amount of oxygen and showed us some postural drainage techniques she hoped would help Ted expel some of the mucus collecting in his lungs. On that Sunday, when most of the world came to a halt in front of the television set, Ted and his plastic tube joined me, my bowl of popcorn, and 129,999,998 others who were watching the Superbowl. Our underdog team, the Broncos, were ahead at the half, but elation didn't last long. We ended up cheering, with most of New England, for the Giants.

It was very hard to persuade Ted to get up and dress himself on Monday morning. Even with oxygen, his breath was coming in gasps; I knew he was much weaker when he didn't have strength to hold up the *Hartford Courant* to read the morning news. At ten the visiting nurse came, and after a brief observation and examination, she announced, "this man is in distress."

She called Dr. Greenglass and described Ted's respiration (44/minute) and the congestion in his lungs. The doctor said he would arrange for an ambulance to bring Ted to his office and would see Ted right away. Within ten minutes the ambulance was at the door, Ted was transferred to it and given an auxiliary oxygen tank, and we were on our way along snow-covered streets. Within fifteen minutes we had driven to the doctor's office where Ted was seen immediately, and within another fifteen minutes we were in the ER at Hartford Hospital. I give these statistics because I was so impressed by the efficiency and the concern that suddenly surrounded us.

After an afternoon of tests and more X rays, Ted was admitted to the eighth floor, and my hospital syndrome, forgotten for four-and-a-half years, was quickly reestablished: the agony of finding a parking place; long waits for the elevator; getting acquainted with nurses, residents, therapists. As I got acquainted with the three other patients in Ted's room, I encountered three different serious problems: diabetes, kidney, heart. How carefree most lives seem when compared with the daily scenarios on a hospital floor. Waves of devotion flow between those walls—from an enthusiastic diabetic adviser to her patient: "Let's get this diet worked out so you can enjoy your meals"; from a soft-voiced nurse carrying messages with her backrubs: "Your daughter called. She is concerned about you"; and from a young doctor's quiet explanation of an angiogram: "I need to know the condition of that carotid artery before we decide to do surgery"—as a concerned wife reaches for the silver-haired patient's hand.

Concern was focused on Ted, too, as he received breathing treatments, electrocardiograms, echocardiographs, tests, tests, and more tests. "I get a lot more rest at home," he complained. He also complained of heartburn, he refused to eat any of the huge meals that were served him, his breathing was still labored, and he developed a temperature. "Oh, that this too too solid flesh would melt," he sighed on a particularly discouraging day.

After ten days of treatments and lots of care from lung specialists and heart doctors, TLC in abundance from his nurses, and constant supervision from Dr. Greenglass, Ted was discharged. His lungs were almost as clear as they had been before his illness, his breathing was

January '87 Setback

almost normal (he needed oxygen only at night), and he seemed on the mend from a siege of bronchitis, pneumonia, viral infection—any or all of the above.

One of Ted's medications was a bronchodilator, Theodur, which he took by mouth. "This is a case of cannibalism!" he remarked drily. When the dosage was reduced to half a tablet a day, Karen consoled him, "Well, in this case half a Theodur is better than a whole Theodur."

"Oh," said Ted thoughtfully, "I wonder if it's better than none."

Sitting in front of the fire, after I came home that first night in January when Ted went to the hospital, I suddenly had an attack of déjà vu. Once again I would have to disappoint Edith, the patient travel agent who, since September, had been spending hours and hours on the phone setting up a schedule for our long-awaited trip to Australia. This time the plans from four years ago were abbreviated because we would be traveling with Ted in a wheelchair, but they still included a tour of New Zealand, and visits to Sydney, Melbourne, Alice Springs, and the Great Barrier Reef. Special hotels had been booked, special seats reserved on the planes. What if we couldn't make it!

There was another reason the very thought of canceling the trip plunged me into despair. When I had outlined this book with the editor, we had agreed that the last chapter would be a journal I would keep of the hazards and opportunities of traveling Down Under in a wheelchair. Could there be a book without that journal? I comforted myself that night in January with the thought that we were not to leave until April 4.

Ted came home from the hospital on February 4 with a good prognosis; we had two months to gain strength. He told everyone about the coming trip, which both of us had looked forward to for so long. We had our pictures taken and we sent for our visas.

By the end of February Ted was off of oxygen completely, so when Karen suggested that he go with them to Philadelphia to spend the weekend with Marcia, we decided it would be a good test for a longer trip. We made a bed in the back of the station wagon for him, and he withstood the trip fairly well. At Marcia's he slept most of the time, but she became well acquainted with my biggest struggle—getting him to eat. Insisting that he was never hungry and that solid food was difficult for him to chew, he subsisted on milk shakes, egg nogs, and hot cereal.

He was tired enough after that weekend for us to decide to cancel the New Zealand part of the trip—the twelve-day tour would be exhausting for him—but we could keep the rest of the plan since it included ten days in Melbourne, where we would be visiting friends and would have rest time. We thought we could safely plan for a shorter trip. After all, if we didn't leave until mid-April, we would have six weeks for improvement.

The image of a yo-yo simply would not leave my mind. It was almost as if one could predict that a good day would be followed by a bad day, a day in which he would not want to get out of bed, would not be interested in reading, would be short of breath with each move. On alternate days, he would wheel himself into the kitchen for breakfast, look at the sports section, and in the evenings, stay up for the MacNeil-Lehrer Report.

"Today I read with both my eyes and ears," he announced proudly early in March, having spent time with Sperber's *Murrow: Life and Times* and *The Portable Dorothy Parker* on Talking Books. But the next day, when I asked about his sighing and groaning, "I do that to prove that I'm still alive."

There was no consistency in our optimism, and to make it more difficult, there were sleepless nights for both of us. How often I quoted to myself Scott Fitzgerald's "Three o'clock in the morning is the midnight of the soul." On one particularly restless night, I started out by reading aloud to Ted an article in the *New Yorker,* "Le Jardin des Plantes," thinking it would remind him of the days we used to walk there, but it was no soporific. In desperation I brought in the tape recorder, and for the next two hours we followed Ishmael and Captain Ahab as they chased a large white whale. I wonder if this could be a footnote in someone's dissertation: innovative uses of *Moby Dick.*

To combat the stay-in-bed syndrome, I brought out carousels of our old color slides to show in the living room: our trips to Greece and the USSR, his visits to Poland, our years in Paris. I noticed that his breathing was easier and more regular when he was diverted, and that was hopeful.

Also hopeful were the things Ted dredged up out of some corner of his mind during the hours he would lie resting in bed. Once, when he had been quiet for a long time, I rushed from upstairs to see if he was all right, planning memorial services all the way to his bedroom. When I got there he opened his eyes, took my hand, and instead of saying "hello" began to recite,

> *Ill fares the land to hastening ills a prey—*
> *Where wealth accumulates and men decay. . . .*

I had been worrying that he was spending those hours worrying about his health; what a relief to know he had been busy calling back words that he had memorized long long ago from Oliver Goldsmith's "The Deserted Village."

One morning I collapsed in laughter as he wheeled himself into the kitchen mumbling,

> *Icarus was a silly cuss,*
> *Him and his daddy Daedalus...*
> *They might of knowed wings made of wax*
> *Couldn't stand sun-heat and hard whacks.*
> *I'd make mine of leather*
> *Or something or other....*

It took our local librarian only ten minutes to call back with the entire poem, "Darius Green and His Flying Machine." I must say I like Ted's version better than John Trowbridge's original:

> *...That Icarus*
>   *Made a Perty muss'*
> *Him an' his daddy Daedalus*
> *They might 'a' knowed wings made o' wax*
> *Wouldn't stand sun-heat an' hard whacks.*
>   *I'll make mine o' luther,*
>   *Ur suthin ur other....*

Those were the good days. At other times, there were visits to Dr. Greenglass after Erin, Ted's faithful and congenial visiting nurse, would discover rales (abnormal respiratory sounds) in Ted's chest. There were days when Ted could not hold his head up for more than half an hour, when he would lie back in bed breathless after putting on his shirt. We had to confront the idea that progress was not steady—that despite the daily use of the nebulizer and the percussor, those lungs, which had been diseased for so long, were working overtime to combat new complications.

January '87 Setback

* * *

While we were fearing it, it came-
But came with less of fear
Because that fearing it so long
Had almost made it fair-

There is a Fitting-a Dismay-
A fitting-a Despair-
'Tis harder knowing it is Due
Than knowing it is Here.

The Trying on the Utmost
The Morning it is new
Is Terribler than wearing it
A whole existence through.

—Emily Dickinson

On a Sunday in March, an unseasonably warm day, I wrote on that day's square on the calendar: "read the *N.Y. Times,* rode my bike, cried a lot." We knew that day that Ted could not be strong enough in one month to make the long, long trip to Australia. I did not have the courage yet to call "Ruth-in-Australia," as we call her to distinguish her from several other Ruth-friends, or to tell Edith, our travel agent, that her hours and hours of arranging had once more been for nothing.

I almost could not bear to pass the "Australia table" in the corner of the bedroom: two envelope-squares of neatly folded travel raincoats, a small white adapter for electric outlets, a newly purchased matched set of plastic-lined cosmetic bags, the half-slip with the clever pocket in the hem for credit cards or traveler's checks, inflatable pillows and tape recordings for the long plane ride, and passports with visas attached.

A good third of one file drawer by my desk was filled with folders marked "Australia" and with letters from our Melbourne friend, Ruth, with plans for each day of our ten-day stay with her. How we were looking forward to hearing the Australia Youth Orchestra, which she helped create and which she has nurtured all these years to bring it to its present place of acclaim in the Australian musical world. I had already given up the dreams of the trip to Rotorua, the Maori Crafts Center, Mt. Cook, Queenstown—all of courageous, independent-minded New Zealand. Now I was having to push out of my mind the white "sails" of the Sydney Opera House, a rose-red Ayers Rock at sunrise, and all those fish in the blue-green waters along the Barrier Reef.

Later, on that decision day, I sat on the deck and tried to contemplate some of the very real discomforts and frustrations we would be avoiding: agonizing decisions about what to pack, piling our luggage onto Ted's lap to get from the baggage claim to the taxi when no porters were to be found, sharing the discomfort of others at the table when Ted choked on food or had a coughing spell, finding a convenient place for him to use his urinal, having to leave him in a strange hotel room if I wanted to take a trip when he was too tired, finding a doctor if his shortness of breath became severe in the middle of the night.

Rationalizations all, but we would gladly have put up with most of those difficulties if Ted had been as strong as he was a year ago—even six months ago.

To be very honest with myself, in the back of my mind was the suspicion that we were succumbing to the path of least resistance, that we were not able "to do it all," that I would be giving up that most subtle of ego trips for the caregiver: "I don't see *how* you do it!" I would have to accept the fact that we are very human, very vulnerable, like everyone else in the world.

The next morning, after breakfast, I climbed the stairs to my sun-filled study-bedroom. Red geraniums and begonias were brilliant, a kolanchoe plant was ready to burst into clusters of small red-orange blossoms, and the crimson butterfly-blooms of the cyclamen hovered over their greenery. I said to myself, as I say every day when I enter this room, "Who in her right mind would ever leave this paradise!" I feel the same when it is sunny, or gray, or snowing, and especially when rain falls quietly against the windows.

And now there will be days to sit on the deck and watch the new rhododendrons flower in the backyard corner where they were planted last summer in memory of our friend who hybridized them. I will have time for the reading that has been neglected during this midwinter siege and time to plant the annuals—to fill the borders with that magnificent boon to those of us who lack green thumbs: impatiens.

And in the bedroom, or reading by his table, or listening to Ed Murrow's "Hear It Now" records, will be Ted, comfortable in his quiet routine, looking forward to the unplanned days as well as the planned ones. And slowly, in the summer's warmth, he will be gaining back his strength.

Ecclesiastes overlooked one juxtaposition: there is a time to do it all, and a time to cease from trying to do it all.

* * *

And the book? What about the book? I had wanted to tell Ted's story not only because it might encourage others, but also because it would be a tribute to his strengths and to his spirit. He had so looked forward to seeing it in book form. Of course, the first part was still a source of wonderment to him—the days he could not remember. Without the Australia trip would there be enough material for a book? I then realized that our own experience was very limited. More knowledge about the medical history of Ted's stroke would be valuable, as well as information about stroke in general. How fortunate we were to have very literate, caring doctors to contribute the chapters that are the appendixes to this volume. Their reports and insights fill a great gap.

Ted's recovery was slow but steady after we decided to cancel our trip.* I worked on the book as he got stronger, and both of us rejoiced in June when he was well enough to fly with Marcia to Green Bay to attend his sixtieth high school reunion. While there, Marcia drove him to the little country cemetery where his grandparents and his mother are buried; they went by the houses where he had lived with his mother while he went to West High School; and in the evening, they hosted a dinner for five cousins and their families.

Our summer days have included a week in Maine with Ted's colleague, "M.E." Fowler, watching the waves crash over Big Boomer, right at our feet. No rock ever had such an appropriate name! In July, we had our fourteenth camping weekend at Tanglewood and later celebrated the golden wedding anniversary of friends on Long Island. A Quaker conference in August was followed by a family trip to bring Bryn home from Horsepower Adventures, her camp in central Pennsylvania. The Wills' new

---

*When we called Ruth-in-Australia on the day in April we were to have arrived in Melbourne, we discovered she had been "in hospital" a week and would be there for some time longer. We could not have carried out some of our plans had we been able to go, after all!

car, "Van Go," proved a very comfortable vehicle for all of us to travel in.

In the mail recently came an announcement from the Smithsonian announcing three-week tours to Australia and New Zealand. We could go in the fall of 1988, visit all the places we had planned to visit twice before, and be going at the right time to enjoy Australia's beautiful spring flowers. Hmmmmmmmmm... why not?

As I hear the sounds from Ted's Talking Book downstairs (Theodore Dreiser's *An American Tragedy*), I think of the many times in the middle of the night, in February and March, when I would creep down to stand at Ted's bedroom door to see if I could see the faintest movement of his covers to let me know he was still breathing. It wouldn't be so out of line to call this story "an American triumph," thanks to the skills and constant caregiving of our doctors, nurses, therapists, aides, and friends.

In the mornings I lie in bed on my sleeping porch listening to Robert J. Lurtsema's birds, singing by radio all the way from Boston, and I realize what competition they have, for they are not the most beautiful sound in my ears when I wake up each day. That most wonderful sound in all the world is the click of the backdoor closing, downstairs. It means that Ted has had a good sleep, has chosen his clothes for the day from his closet and dressed himself, has wheeled into the kitchen, opened the backdoor to get the *Hartford Courant,* closed the door, and is now reaching for the sports section.

No symphony, no chorus, no birdsong can equal that eloquent click.

CHAPTER XIII

Coping

That Love is all there is,
Is all we know of Love;
It is enough, the freight should be
Proportioned to the groove.
   —*Emily Dickinson*

The subject for the discussion group at Quaker Meeting that day had been "Suffering." On the way home Ted was silent for a few blocks and then said, thoughtfully, "I suppose most of the people in that room think I have suffered a lot since I had my stroke. I don't think I have suffered, either physically or mentally. I don't feel that way at all. A lot of bad things have happened in my life but I've never suffered, really."

"That's one reason you've been able to adjust to this as well as you have," I said. "How did you get that attitude? It's one I admire a lot."

"I think I got it from my mother," he said quietly.

Grace Boyden Paullin was a special kind of heroine, I realized, as I thought of the problems she had coped with. Raised in a small farming community in Wisconsin, she began teaching after eight years of schooling, as I mentioned earlier. A few years later, when teaching in Green Bay, she met and married the Baptist minister. In 1917, Ted's father went as a volunteer with the YMCA to France. There he fell in love with a woman with whom he worked, and after the war, he returned to Milwaukee, his last pastorate, long enough to settle his affairs. He then entered law school at the University of Chicago, leaving the ministry and his family behind. Ten-year-old Theodore never saw him again.

"It must have been terribly hard for your mother to face the stigma of divorce in those days and to have full responsibility for you, besides," I said.

"Oh yes," Ted agreed quickly. "And she had no money at all. My father was supposed to send her some for my support—about fifteen dollars a month, I think—but that stopped after a few months. In all those years I never heard my mother feel sorry for herself, not once. I guess that's why I don't think I have suffered particularly, because I've never felt sorry for myself, either."

"That's a pretty fine legacy," I said.

But not feeling sorry for yourself doesn't mean there may not be very painful regrets. A group of us were talking about our favorite and least favorite words or phrases. After I'd said that the words that make me cringe are "to kill time" and the words that make my spirit soar are "no problem," Ted contributed his. "I can't stand the word *irregardless*," he said, and he was reminded that on that very day, a Supreme Court justice had reprimanded a lawyer appearing before him for using that same nonword.

"But what is your favorite?" I listened as eagerly as the others.

"My favorite words are 'Let's take a walk' because I can't," he said.

I was reminded of Emily Dickinson once more:

> *Water, is taught by thirst.*
> *Land—by the Oceans passed.*

Ted hadn't spoken in a tone of self-pity; it was just a

sad statement of fact. I only hope I have that same kind of strength if someday I'm unable to walk.

I realize that the legacies from my father and mother are quite different, but my parents, too, like Grace Paullin, taught by example rather than by exhortation.

From my father I inherited an insatiable curiosity. (No plane trip was ever made by my Dad without a visit to the cockpit to find out the amount of fuel being used, miles per hour, years of pilot's service and his place of birth, etc.) In our childhood Dad instigated many contests: who could find the campus tree with the largest circumference? who could identify the most items under a large napkin, which was lifted for only a second? who could give the proper names for the cloud formations? who could recite the Presbyterian catechism first? who could write the best journal (a requirement after any excursion or vacation trip)?

From my mother I absorbed a sort of compulsive compassion (part of her Cherokee heritage?). I remember several Thanksgiving dinners that were delayed because she had to drive across town to take a meal to a widowed elderly friend before we could have our turkey. Mother was obsessed, too, with the history of Manhattan, Kans. (her mother and father had graduated from Kansas State in 1888). As a result of her persistent endeavors, a beautiful stone house from pioneer days was preserved and given to the state as a museum. Her determination (called by some just plain stubbornness) influenced us all. My share of it was sometimes evident, to the dismay of some, in the days that followed Ted's illness. In that autumn in 1982 after his stroke, if an interviewer had asked that television standard, "What did you *feel* about this event?" I would have had the same answer Jeana Yeager had after her trip around the world in the Voyager: "I was just too busy to feel."

Coping

I have often thought that going through a traumatic experience such as the critical period of Ted's sudden stroke and hospitalization is much like being in a theatrical production. You have to be on stage every day; you are not allowed to let down or be ill or "goof off"; you become, for a short time, the center of attention of friends and relatives. When it comes right down to it, the caregivers, as well as the actors, need almost unlimited supplies of adrenalin and stamina for the "run of the show."

The central "given" for both the caregiver and the one being cared for is that *there are no options*. Survival is all, so you might as well take it in good humor and make the best of it. I guess making the best of it, for me, comes with the genes. When the Slinky we had as kids got damaged so it wouldn't slink down the stairway anymore, my mother sprayed it with gilt paint, mounted it on a gilded cardbord box, and used it to file her letters.

This is certainly not to say that the life of the caregiver runs a smooth course. A friend, writing once about her invalid husband, described my experiences exactly: "I cannot show frustration even though he expresses great frustration; I need to adjust constantly to his moods and needs; I must be willing, cheerfully, to stop whatever I am doing at any moment to answer his call. But how grateful I am," she adds, "to have him!"

To give up the luxury of becoming angry is a real deprivation. Sometimes when I hear "Shut the door," "Give me the paper," "Turn off the light," or "Get me the sugar," I feel like shouting "I am not a servant." But on one occasion when I did express my frustration, Ted said, in his broken voice, "But when I say 'shut the door,' it's not like when other people say it." I realize that it is an economy of language, not a command, and my anger dissolves in a hurry.

When I was tired and frustrated a couple of times and did blow up, the consequences for Ted were not worth the price of my outlet. He crumpled completely. Of course, there are many times *he* must resent being told what to do, having his schedule for the day outlined by someone else, being totally dependent on others for errands, being nagged to eat and to exercise. How often must he want to scream, "I am not a child!"

Both of us have had to face and accept new limitations and deprivations.

A minimum of self-pity, lots of inquisitiveness, compassion, and persistence—in addition to these "legacies," I have often thought about what in our early environment has helped us in these post-stroke years.

The era in which we grew up is, of course, one of the big influences. There is a preoccupation prevalent today with which Ted and I were completely unfamiliar: we had no time to spend on introspection. We were so busy making ends meet economically that we didn't stop to ask "Who am I?" or to wonder whether we were happy. In the long run, the less we strived for happiness, the more we seemed to find it. Despite our inalienable right, as proclaimed in the Declaration of Independence, we did not pursue it, but how we did enjoy it when it turned out to be a by-product of our activities.

If there is such a word as *extrospection,* it would describe the focus of our energies: we constantly questioned, not ourselves, but what we perceived as the aspects of our society that fall short of our ideals of a good life for all; and always, in the foreground, was our desire for a world at peace. Marcia and I stood in the first Quaker vigil that formed a line around the Pentagon in 1960. Ted, Karen, Marcia, and I marched in Washington in 1966 to protest the war in Vietnam, leading Marcia to paraphrase a slogan in use at the time, "The family that pickets together stickets together." When the misfortunes of the world loom so large, one sees one's own misfortunes in perspective. Perhaps that has stood us in good stead—that, and resilience.

In our youth, resilience was taken for "granite" (a fortuitous misspelling in a letter from a friend): we were taught that it was a solid, steadfast commodity we could count on. It was all around us. We counted the tombstones of children in pioneer cemeteries, added up the hours some of us worked to get an education during the Depression, considered the thousands of lost jobs, lost homes, and lost hopes in those years. Elasticity, flexibility, buoyancy—all were necessary to survive.

Marguerite Yourcenar said once, "If you can say 'mad with joy' you should be able to say 'wise with grief.'" We have enjoyed that kind of "madness," and we keep on trying to achieve a measure of wisdom!

Once more, Emily Dickinson:

> *We never know how high we are*
> *Till we are asked to rise*
> *And then if we are true to plan*
> *Our statures touch the skies-*

We always hoped that coping would be part of our plan, but no one, *no one* ever said that being true to that plan would be easy.

We grow accustomed to the Dark-
When Light is put away-
As when the Neighbor holds the Lamp
To witness her Goodbye-

A Moment-We uncertain step
For newness of the night-
Then-fit our Vision to the Dark-
And meet the Road-erect-

And so of larger-Darknesses-
Those Evenings of the Brain-
When not a Moon disclose a sign-
Or Star-come out-within-

The Bravest-grope a little-
And sometimes hit a Tree
Directly in the Forehead-
But as they learn to see-

Either the Darkness alters-
Or something in the sight
Adjusts itself to Midnight-
And Life steps almost straight.

—Emily Dickinson

Afterwords

by Ted's Two Doctors

Afterwords

Ted's Hospitalization: A Physician's Retrospective

Arthur D. Wolf, M.D.

I remember it well. It was a Monday night. I had just arrived home, about ten o'clock, when the call came from my answering service: "Ted Paullin has been found unconscious in his car and taken to the emergency room at Hartford Hospital. His wife wants you there."

It sounded ominous although I have learned over the years that a hasty diagnosis on the basis of cryptic information often turns out to be a misdiagnosis on direct observation. But, as usual in such situations, my mind started running through my own "data bank," conjuring up relevant knowledge I could apply to the specifics of Ted's case once I learned them, and planning ahead for diagnostic evaluation, management, and treatment. I knew from experience that this could be a fruitless exercise, for it was not uncommon, once I arrived at the hospital, to find the patient's condition altogether different from what I'd expected; indeed, sometimes the patient would be up and walking around.

Nevertheless, as I drove to the hospital—as fast as the law and prudence would allow—the old habit held. I did not know Ted as his physician, and therefore I had little clinical history to draw on. But as a friend of twenty-five years, I knew something of the medical events of his life. That he was a cigarette smoker for a long time I was well aware. That he had quit several years before had both surprised and delighted me, as it had most of his other friends. That he persisted with a chronic cough that sounded deep and productive of sputa was, alas, still evident when one was in his presence. I vaguely knew that special X-ray exams several years ago had shown bronchiectasis, a disorder in which a number of medium-sized bronchi (air tubes much like branches of a tree) have widened, lost some of their natural elasticity, and allowed the pooling of secretions and inhaled pollutants and organisms. In this setting, pulmonary infections and chronic cough are more common and harder to manage. Any illness affecting voluntary control of respiration and prolonging recumbency was likely to create problems in a person with this disorder. Ted was to be no exception.

The other thing running through my mind was more personal than medical. As I had known him, Ted's sense of personal worth lay in his mind and spirit, not so much in his body. Though limited now in physical tolerance by his pulmonary status, he had never been a "jock." His principal chosen physical exercise now was dancing with his wife on special occasions, and this he did very well. Philosophically, he abhorred any notion that "might makes right" and espoused "mind over matter" in his political and religious views. Although to be rendered unconscious is devastating for anybody, whatever the cause, I knew that, for Ted, recovery would be tolerable to the degree that any impairment was more of the body than of the cognitive mind. (The locus of spirit is not anatomically defined, though I suspect it is both inside and outside and all around both of these.) Thus, the cause of Ted's "unconsciousness" was of utmost importance in prognosticating in what ways and to what degree he would be able to function, physically and mentally, in the future.

It is obvious that the word *unconscious* describes a mental state of low awareness and responsiveness. The primary cause, however, may not reside in the brain. A fall in blood pressure due to cardiac standstill (no electrical impulse) or dysrhythmia (insufficient coordinated contraction) may lead to an insufficient flow of oxygenated blood to the brain, thereby resulting in such a malfunction. Toxins, be they chemicals or gases (e.g., barbiturates or carbon monoxide gas), may lead to such a state. A sudden blow to the brain may alter electrical activity and leave the victim unconscious. But for anyone of Ted's age, the most common cause would probably be a disruption in intracranial circulation. This could be a blockage in an artery by a clot, thus preventing the flow of blood to the area served by that artery. Or it could be a leakage from an artery (a hemorrhage) with the blood pushing aside brain cells and disrupting their normal function and connections. The physiologic response to either event would soon involve the mechanisms of inflammatory repair. Such a process involves the dilation of small blood vessels in the area, and the passage of fluid and scavenger cells across capillary walls. The net result is swelling. This doesn't constitute much of a problem if the original injury is in a place with space to expand, such as the skin. However, in the cranial cavity, essentially a closed box, such expansion seriously compresses adjacent structures, leading to potentially severe malfunctions in cells not initially directly involved. Thus, with the passage of time and accumulation of such edema (fluid), the clinical picture may worsen.

So it was that I speculated as I drove on, assuming that the apparent suddenness of the event probably meant that Ted had had a vascular accident involving his brain directly. The location and extent and type of this accident would determine the prognosis, but only in statistical terms. Just as important—qualitatively rather than quantitatively—was the individual to whom this had happened. For as the quintessential savant of American (and later, British) medicine, Sir William Osler, wrote, it's "much more important to know what sort of patient has a disease than to know what sort of disease a patient has." Ted was a person (now apparently a patient) to whom cognitive powers were a unique and special marker of his particular worth (without negating the worth of other powers in other persons). What would be his status when I arrived?

This is what I found: Ted had arrived in the ER in a comatose state, initially unresponsive to stimuli. His respirations were described as "agonal," a term often applied to the pattern of breathing noted in individuals in a near-death condition. Though his blood pressure was normal (130/70), his pulse was rapid (116) and sometimes irregular. His pupils were small, the right being 3 mm, the left 2 mm in diameter. His limbs were flaccid. The plantar reflexes (evoked by scratching the soles of his feet) indicated an abnormality affecting his brain.

The initial treatment was to establish ways of controlling vital functions. He was intubated (a tube with an inflatable cuff near its end is passed via the mouth between the vocal cords and into the trachea) to provide a means of controlling the passage of gases (oxygen in and carbon dioxide out) through his lungs. An intravenous line was inserted so both fluids and drugs could be introduced into his circulation. Because the profundity of his altered consciousness suggested the accumulation of edema fluid in his brain, he was given an injection of Decadron, a cortisonelike drug that helps decrease edema in the inflammatory response.

It seemed to help, for within a few hours he was improved. He was described as awake (he couldn't talk because of the endotracheal tube in his larynx), could respond with a hand squeeze on request, and was moving his left arm and leg spontaneously. However, there were no facial movements or eye movements in certain directions when requested; his plantar reflexes were still clearly abnormal; and although his pupils responded reflexly to light, they were still contracted. The neurologist who had now come in to see him gave his impression: "A cerebellar hemorrhage with resultant swelling and compression of adjacent tissue!"

The next step was to confirm this, localize it, and consider what immediate treatment was indicated. Ted was taken to the radiology unit where a CT scan was done. This process, relatively new in radiology, has revolutionized diagnosis in relatively inaccessible parts of the body. Essentially, it allows a doctor to obtain cross-sectional views through contrasting tissues with different densities, without disturbing these tissues in any way. When used to examine the brain, a CT scan is comparable to taking the brain out of the cranial cavity, cutting across it in any direction, looking at the cut surface for any change in structure, and then reassembling it and placing it back in the skull as if nothing had ever happened to it!

The CT diagnosis: "A cerebellar bleed in the region of the left dentate nucleus with questionable compression of the pons."

The cerebellum is in the hind brain. A small, fistlike structure looking rather like a cauliflower head, it is essential for the proper timing of muscular action in coordinated activity. It has connections with the front part of the brain where impulses to move certain muscles arise (the so-called motor cortex). It also connects with certain specialized collections of cells in the brain stem that govern and coordinate a number of more discrete functions, as well as the descending tracts of nerves carrying messages from the motor cortex to distant parts of the body.

This whole system is highly organized to provide smooth, finely tuned motions with innumerable messages to contract certain muscles a little, a lot, or some amount in between. At the same time, other muscles, in opposition to that action, must relax a little, a lot, or some amount in between. If it were not for such integration, your simple command to your hand to touch your eyelid might sent your fist crashing unchecked into your eye. Or the advancing of one leg forward in your gait might throw your whole body to the ground with the momentum of that action. In lesions of the cerebellum there is a prolongation of the interval between the motor command and the following triphasix motor sequence involving coordination of opposing muscle groups. The dentate nucleus in the cerebellum is a specialized collection of cells receiving inhibitory fibers from another region of the cerebellar cortex (outermost part). It dampens the normal physiologic tremor that would occur if alternating contractions/relaxations of muscle groups were not smoothly and rapidly sending messages back and forth as to their actions. Consider how a simple reaching out for some object would appear if each motion extending your hand had to be checked for location before proceeding to a little more extension. It would appear as a staccatolike jerkiness rather than a steady flowing stream.

The consequences of a cerebellar lesion in human beings do not always respect the neat boundaries established by the laboratory experiments of neuroanatomists in working with closely related species. But the net effect is the same. There's a loss of muscle tone, reduced coordination of volitional movements, minor muscular weakness, increased fatigability, decreased equilibrium, and impaired associated movements. Most if not all these consequences awaited Ted—if he survived!

And what to do to ensure that he did survive the immediate consequences of this cerebello-vascular accident? The pons is a critical area in the brain stem, the focal point where many nerve fibers come together and pass down to the spinal cord. It is also the site of some specialized centers of control of respiration and heart rate. Pressure on it can lead to profound disruption of those functions and even death. The compression of brain tissue by a continuing hemorrhage mandates measures to establish the site and arrest the bleeding.

Fortunately, a cerebellar hemorrhage is one of the few vascular calamities of the brain treatable by surgery. To stop the bleeding and relieve the pressure on adjacent tissues not only can be life saving, but also can limit the extent of ultimate residual damage in a surviving person. In Ted's case, immediate surgery seemed to be imperative, a judgment confirmed by the neurosurgeon we called in after the CT scan had been interpreted. The operating room was alerted, and soon Ted was on his way to the first of a number of operations that would ensue in the coming weeks.

The operative note, as I read it later, can be succinctly stated. A hole was made through Ted's skull, just below the hairline in the back of his head on the left. A clot beneath the covering of his brain was removed. An incision was made into the cerebellum. In the region of the dentate nucleus, another clot was suctioned out. In the depth of this wound there was "brisk bleeding" from an artery. This was coagulated with the application of high heat from a special instrument. In all, 25 to 50 cc (five to ten teaspoons) of blood were evacuated. The covering (dura mater) was replaced, the hole in the skull repaired, and Ted was off to the neurosurgical intensive care unit.

So far it had been high drama, especially for his family—and for me, as well. The surgical intervention had probably saved Ted's life, but before he left the hospital there would be repeated threats to his survival and ultimate recovery. Still to appear were other specialists in pulmonary medicine, urology, infectious disease, ENT (ear, nose, and throat), nutrition, and surgery, not to mention a vast supporting cast of nurses, resident physicians, respiratory therapists, physical therapists, social workers, and so on. Shunted to the sidelines in the first few hours, his family was to reenter the scenario and play a major role in the evolution of his recovery—its ups and downs from one stage to the next, with intervening crises and setbacks. But the major character, center stage, was to remain Ted Paullin—"down but not out."

The human body has wonderful, purposeful reflexes that serve to protect it in almost all ways. We blink to avoid dust in our eyes, sneeze and cough to expel pollutants, withdraw a hand or leg from sharp objects, and push away from our body anything causing discomfort, pressure, or pain. Most people will allow their bodies to be invaded by needles and instruments when they understand the reasons. But when such understanding is beclouded by altered mental states, the primitive reflexes of warding off perceived bodily threats take over. Hence the frequent challenge, especially to the nursing staff, to prevent patients from reflexly removing from their bodies the innumerable tubes and lines that deliver essential fluids, chemicals, drugs, or oxygen, or that remove wastes and other drainage. Such primitive reflexes also often lead patients to attempt to remove themselves, unattended, from a bed or chair, thus incurring the danger of falls as well as disconnecting vital lines and tubes. Patients cannot always understand this, and families, out of compassion and sometimes pressure from the patient, are often unwitting accomplices in "liberating" them. To prevent such occurrences, the ideal solution is to have trained medical personnel constantly in attendance, but logistics and economics do not always allow this. Hence the frequent necessity to restrain a patient physically by other measures—for instance, with ties to the bed or with vests that can be attached to a bed or chair; with the restriction of physical space; with chemical sedation; or with the voice or hands of an attendant or family member. Physicians and nurses would not themselves like to be "tied down," and they impose it on patients only reluctantly. But even then this does not always suffice, and Ted was to be no exception as to both need and lack of success.

His operation was in the early hours of September 21. In the ICU, he was noted to be awake, moving all four extremities. The tube into his trachea was removed (extubation), and respiratory therapy involving intermittent positive pressure of air/oxygen was started to be sure he was inspiring sufficiently to ensure good oxygenation of his lungs and tissues. Later that day, however, he developed an increasingly labored respiratory effort, and the endotracheal tube had to be reinserted. He was able to follow some simple commands, but alas, he didn't follow all commands! He pulled out the catheter that had been placed in his bladder to ensure that he didn't retain urine and to provide an accurate measure of kidney function. When the resident couldn't get the tube back in, a urologist was called, who reinserted it successfully.

Because of the respiratory problems requiring reintubation, a pulmonary specialist saw Ted the next day. His impression was that the immediate problem was acute upper airway obstruction, possibly complicated by nasal bleeding and the accumulation of blood farther down. The endotracheal tube was to be repositioned, and later Ted was to be reevaluated for extubation.

On the 23rd, Ted was less arousable, clearly an ominous sign. Another CT scan of the brain was done, which showed a hydrocephalus—an accumulation, beyond normal volume, of fluid in one of the ventricles (fluid cavities) of the brain. This required the insertion of a tube, which was then left in place, into this ventricle to allow drainage of excess fluid and prevent compression of adjacent brain tissue.

By the 24th it was apparent that respirations on his own were unlikely to occur yet. The endotracheal tube would have to be removed. The continued pressure against the lining of the throat and trachea from the inflated cuff eventually causes erosion of this mucous surface and therefore cannot be left in for more than a few days. A tracheotomy—an opening into the trachea below the level of the vocal cords—provides a means of delivering air under controlled circumstances to the lungs. Equally important because the vocal cords are then bypassed, thus preventing an effective cough, it also provides access to the trachea and lungs to suction out secretions that might block air from reaching deeper into the lungs. So on this day a tracheotomy was performed by an ENT consultant, who at the same time examined

A Physician's Retrospective

the nasal passages for bleeding. He found more than usual, but not enough to be a major problem.

The placing of the tracheotomy and the tube in this opening enabled better control of the secretion in Ted's lungs. But again, there were his chronic lung problems to take into account. Unable to move around, not aware enough to try to cough, and with secretions pooling in parts of the lungs too deep to suction, he was a sitting duck for serious lung infection. By the 27th he was described as having increased amounts of thick yellow-gray sputa being suctioned. His lungs sounded juicier when heard through a stethoscope. The measurement of oxygen and carbon dioxide dissolved in his blood showed he was getting less of the former and retaining too much of the latter. His color was more cyanotic (blue). He was more lethargic, and now another chest X ray showed bilateral infiltrates (pneumonia on both sides). Bacteriologic culture of his sputa showed an organism, *Seriatia marcescens,* and he was placed on appropriate antibiotics.

He seemed stabilized for a while, but fever persisted. It was apparent that the battle had shifted from his brain to his lungs. He was not awake enough or alert enough to cough effectively. Suddenly, on October 5, he stopped breathing, and his blood pressure dropped to 80 mm Hq systolic. He was immediately connected to the nearby respirator, and soon after he began to have spontaneous respirations. By the next day he could be weaned off the respirator easily.

At the same time, he was noted to have a significant amount of discharge around his trachea. It was thought this might be a source of infection and continuing fever. The latter might also be secondary to the antibiotic (Ancef) that he was receiving (a so-called drug fever). He was switched to a different antibiotic (Nafcillin). A subsequent rash developed, possibly related to the antibiotics. What system of the body was to be spared?

And what of the rest of his body? The fuels we have stored up do not last indefinitely. Simple existence even in an unresponsive state requires baseline caloric expenditure. The presence of infection and fever increases this demand. Altered consciousness affects our ability to chew and swallow even though we do this reflexly to a certain degree. A cerebellar lesion can seriously impair the coordinated activity necessary to get food to go down the esophagus to the stomach and not down the trachea to the lungs. The body needs more than the glucose, sodium, potassium, and water provided in the usual intravenous fluids. After the first week, Ted had been started on feedings of greater caloric variety and amount through a tube placed through the nose, down the esophagus, and into the stomach. This was yet another "invading irritant," to be reflexly plucked out if he could get his hands on it. And he did—repeatedly.

The nutrition consultant noted in the first week of October that Ted's fat stores were decreased, his muscle masses generally reduced, and the blood tests of serum albumin and transferrin were very low, indicating early protein and caloric malnutrition despite the tube feedings. In this situation a gastrostomy (an opening through the abdominal wall directly into the stomach) is often done to provide direct access to the gastrointestinal tract and get rid of the nasogastric feeding tube. But in the presence of infection in the body this involves more risk, so it was deferred until he was better and no longer receiving the antibiotics. In addition, there was now a concern, expressed first on the 8th, that Ted's continuing fever and greatly elevated blood sedimentation rate might indicate subacute bacterial endocarditis (an infection of the heart valves, sometimes occurring with prolonged infections elsewhere in the body, especially if resistance is low with malnutrition). Fortunately, an echocardiogram (made by sound waves that can quantitate shape and thickness by bouncing off structures) showed that structurally the valves appeared normal.

As the weeks went by, the battlefield increasingly became his nutritional status, and he was given additional nutrients intravenously. As helpful as that treatment was, however, it didn't allow natural processes, through digestive enzymes in the gastrointestinal tract, to break down all the essential foods into the basic compounds necessary for the body. And, of course, it bypassed the liver as the major chemical processing plant receiving raw materials from the intestinal tract via the portal circulation. (This is a one-way highway by which normally all assimilated foodstuffs pass on their way into the body for further refinement and then storage or distribution.)

While his doctors waited until it was safe to do the gastrostomy and thus get rid of the nasogastric tube that was so terribly annoying, the daily challenge became retention of this tube. Ted's hands were wrapped, mitten-fashion, in bandages so that he couldn't grasp the tube to pull it out. Since this didn't always suffice because he could somehow work the tube out anyway, his mittened hands were then tied to the sides of the bed (or chair, as he was beginning to be placed in one for intervals each day). But even this was not always enough! The almost primitive ability of human beings to disengage themselves from restraints suggests some Houdini-like genes in the least of us. It's a constant source of amazement and frustration to medical personnel—witness the progress note in his chart: "Seems impossible to keep feeding tube in place." This was on October 25, after many previous days of notes about replacing the tube almost daily.

The joy at proceeding to do a gastrostomy on the 26th was felt by many. For Ted, the obvious relief was in no longer having the constant awareness of a tube in his nose and throat. His family could share in that. But I'm also aware of the relief for the nurses, who were responsible twenty-four hours a day for ensuring that their patients maintained all tubes in place. And finally, the resident physicians no longer had the unpleasant task of reinserting a nasogastric tube into a patient who often reflexly fought the insertion. It's hard enough in a patient whose swallowing coordination is intact and who therefore makes it easier with coaching to get the tube down into the esophagus and not into the trachea. Imagine what it's like in a patient with cerebellar dysfunction, who has difficulty swallowing a simple sip of water without some of it going the wrong way and into the lungs!

But it's a mistake to think a gastrostomy operation solves all problems. The gastrointestinal tract has evolved (as in other biological beings) to meet our species' specific needs. We are both carnivores and herbivores. The sight, smell, and taste of foods we need and like can begin to turn on increased production, and then secretion, of digestive enzymes in the stomach, pancreas, and small intestines to break down the foods when they reach these organs. Chewing induces secretion of salivary enzymes, which also begin acting on carbohydrates while still in the mouth. We govern the rate of intake through the mouth both consciously and unconsciously. When all these stimuli are bypassed by direct introduction of foods into the stomach, the result is not always the nice physiologic response the body is designed to make. A more usual response is an increased transit time of food and secretions down through the intestines. This means decreased time for absorption of nutrients as well as for reabsorption of water. The latter process is the means by which we package our wastes to become a solid for delivery at the farthest end. The net result of frequent increased transit times is both malnutrition and dehydration, all as a consequence of what is commonly called diarrhea.

To obviate some of these problems, the infusion of foods (usually in a liquid form) is performed at a slow rate (either by gravity or by a manual push, as with a large syringe or an infusion pump). The supervision and monitoring of this process take time; therefore, the ultimate goal is to achieve intermittent feedings, much as we do in our natural state. To "train" the GI tract to do this without rebelling is no simple task. After all, it sometimes acts like it has a mind of its own, as when it reacts to thoughts and feelings—to wit, "a nervous stomach." But our largely nonthinking, noncognitive gut can learn.

Ted had had some problems with nasogastric feedings. The day before the gastrostomy was done, the nutritionist wrote, "This patient is obviously nutritionally depleted." He was putting out less urine via his urinary catheter, and his BUN (blood urea nitrogen) was rising, which also indicated dehydration despite intravenous fluids. The day after the gastrostomy, no sounds of bowel function were heard—not uncommon after any abdominal surgery. But by the following day, feedings via the gastrostomy could be started, and within a few days it was noted that diarrhea had slowed. Five days later it was possible to remove the indwelling tube from the opening and begin the intermittent introduction of a tube and feeding six times a day. He was on his way to a more "human" (read "tubeless") existence!

Of course, the tracheotomy tube was still in place, and it was still a concern. The difficulty in coordinating swallowing so that liquids and solids only went down the esophagus was still a mark of his initial cerebellar injury. Our lungs are designed to absorb gases, not liquids or solids. When the trap door (epiglottis) doesn't close properly over the larynx (which, with the vocal cords, is the entrance to the trachea), these substances will enter the lungs. This may happen by direct force (swallowing or vomiting), by gravity, or during the inspiration of air. Their presence in the lungs will provoke a reaction of several sorts. It may be chemical, as with gastric juices, which are meant to break down food, not lung surfaces. It may be infectious, due to organisms in the mouth and throat. In either case it causes an inflammatory response called pneumonia. Having anything other than air sucked into the lungs is called aspiration. Such a pneumonia is therefore designated as "aspiration pneumonia." The severity of it varies, but it can be very difficult to treat. It is a constant threat when swallowing mechanisms are altered by disease or drugs, as with anesthesia.

This was still a problem for Ted. Though he was not fed solids or liquids by mouth, his saliva still had to go someplace, and preferably *not* down into the trachea. The plastic trach tube was still in place, with a cuff inside the trachea usually inflated to prevent aspiration. An occasional sip of clear water was tried to see if Ted could swallow it correctly. Examination of his throat reflexes by stimulating the back of his pharynx under direct observation continued to show a poor gag reflex (thus poor coordination of the normal response). On October 15, one physician raised the question in the chart of "a change from the cuff tube to a metal trach, if not aspirating." The next note—same day, different person—stated (almost in anger, it seemed), "But he is aspirating!

Tracheotomy tubes can be covered with a finger on the outside so that, with the cuff deflated, air exhaled from the lungs will exit through the larynx and mouth rather than directly to the outside via the tube. This permits verbal expression in a comprehensible fashion though not exactly a natural voice. It's tiring. It involves coordination, covering the tube when speaking, and then uncovering it to get a maximal inhalation of air back into the lungs. By early November Ted was aspirating very little so that there was no longer a need for a cuff, and by the 10th it seemed appropriate to change him to a metal trach tube. In addition to the fact that the metal tube was less irritating to the trachea, it also made conversation easier.

Though he was still having copious secretions that could be suctioned from his lungs via the trach tube, he could still have the tube plugged for long periods of time and breathe comfortably through his upper airway. Nature intended that the air reaching our lungs first be warmed and humidified—hence, the ingenious system of baffles (rather like fins of a radiator) in the nose. In addition, the mucous membrane covering those turbinates (the baffles) in the nose may also trap dust, germs, and other pollutants. If air is taken directly from the outside through a trach tube, this advantage is lost. Although it can be compensated for by mechanically introducing filtered, warm, moist air directly into the trach from special apparatus, that requires one more annoying appendage attached to the patient. What a joy, then, to shuck off another tether and be able to breathe through the normal route most of the time!

There was still one tube of which to be rid. The urinary catheter, attached to a drainage bag, is perhaps the least cumbersome of all the tubes. But it is an annoying irritant to the mucous membrane of the urethra, and it is a possible route by which bacteria may enter the bladder and initiate infections that can spread throughout the body. The conscious control of excretion of urine from the bladder is one of the conditioned (learned) reflexes that the body often loses following any insult to the brain. Retraining the bladder is not as simple a case of "mind over matter" as it might seem. Both learning not to allow the bladder to empty reflexly at any time (or place) and learning to empty the bladder when it is moderately full now became old habits for Ted to reestablish. By early November, with the retention catheter removed, he was voiding reflexly when urine accumulated in his bladder. But he didn't empty the bladder completely each time, and he was not aware of the sensation of voiding. Intermittent catheterizations, done just after voiding, showed residual volumes up to a cup of urine. Medication (urecholine) was added, and over the next few weeks it was charted that he "appears to be regaining some control" and therefore continence.

The story so far has been so involved with the primitive functions of breathing, coughing, voiding, and eating that one might wonder whether any attention was paid to the activities of daily living by which we distinguish human beings. When we think of rehabilitation following a stroke, the image is usually of physical therapists teaching a person to walk again. That too became an important part of Ted's program. Unlike the more common strokes, in which voluntary control on one side of the forebrain is affected, Ted's illness involved primarily the coordination of function, which was much harder to regain. While he was still hospitalized, it was noted that "after intensive physical therapy, attempts at ambulation were unsuccessful." He even made one attempt, unsolicited and unsupervised, to get out of bed alone one night. He fell but was uninjured. Nonetheless, there were enough gains, hopes, and family support to believe that Ted would continue to improve with further rehab so that he could eventually make it home. And who knows, after that! So plans were made, application submitted, and acceptance granted for transfer to Jefferson House. This is a specialized geriatric facility of Hartford Hospital, where the emphasis is on continuing independence in functional gains, leading to life at a lesser level of need for care. That magic day, not foreseen some eight-and-a-half weeks before, finally came, and on November 19 Ted took one more giant step forward.

* * *

As I reflect now on this portion of his story, of this stroke in this person, many facets stand out. It's a little miracle, all its own, as it is for countless people in the stories of their struggles, hopes, failures, and successes. It's a four-part story that involves *self* and *others,* each on two levels. The most basic level is at the simple magic of the human body. By no means infallible, subject at times to self-destruct, inevitably drawn to fail at the end, it is so magnificently capable of adjusting to insult and injury by compensation and repair that it is truly one of the greatest wonders of all creation. Hence the wisdom of another savant of medicine, one of a more ancient time. As Hippocrates wrote, "The human body is the physician of its own illnesses."

But even that great "physician" may benefit from

help. Ted's survival and recovery were enhanced and aided by a host of individuals, and with them the modern accoutrements of their trade. The panoply of players on this stage was vast, some with major, some with minor roles. In looking back I'm impressed not just with the number of specialized, dedicated persons with skills, but also at what those skills themselves represent: the accumulation of knowledge, developed and transmitted over many decades from many people. Those persons are the silent, unseen players, not glimpsed on stage nor credited in the program, but whose contributions to the scenario are just as real. The complexity of modern medicine, the multiplicity of its specialized practitioners, and the seeming distancing of the patient by all the machinery seems to diminish the personal attention of an earlier time and place of practice. But the traditions of professionalism are still there, and the apparent reliance on cold, hard data is met and well balanced by warm and caring hands and heart.

Ted's body itself was involved in his healing, as were other people, those with medical and nursing skills. But it can be argued that, even with the services available to him in this highly developed and respected hospital, he might not have survived without the loving care and skills of his family. From the earliest moments, and for weeks of which he has no conscious recall, his wife and daughters were there—talking to him, reading to him, playing music on tapes for him, stroking and caressing him. We know that some animals in infancy may wither and die without the touch, warmth, and sound of their parent. The same may be true for humans. But even such physical nurturing is not enough if the emotional needs are not met. Is it not then equally possible that adults in mentally confused, even nonconscious states may re-

A Physician's Retrospective

spond in a like manner to nurture? Good nurses (alas, more often than many doctors) know this and act accordingly. Of course, many families do likewise. I'm convinced that this may be the most important ingredient in survival, and then in recovery to whatever extent, for most people. It may not always be enough, but what a powerful force it is when it is present. This total story bears abundant testimony to that.

And finally, the fourth level in this epic is that of Ted's character and spirit. My earliest thoughts while driving to the hospital that September night were a foretaste of what was to come. That part of the brain devoted to reason and meaning rather than to coordination was spared, and with it the grandeur of Ted's recovery was made possible. The stimulation of those things that meant most to him—family, music, thought, meaning— was there for him from the beginning, making life worth living despite the loss of many physical powers. Autumn was about to begin when tragedy struck. Winter was to come without any assurance that the spring of heart and mind would follow for him. His mental status in the early weeks was described as "fluctuating—sometimes alert, sometimes confused, sometimes nodding appropriately in response to questions, sometimes hallucinating." With some regained consciousness but an inability to speak with the earlier trach tubes still in, he used a pad and pencil to communicate and used them avidly. For an extremely verbal man, this was most important. It meant that language, so necessary to him for communication, was still his to command. And witness this note in the chart, one month after admission: "Quite alert and bright. Enthusiastically conducting music played on his bedside tape deck" (probably with his hands swathed in bandage mittens to prevent removal of a tube—how I'd like a picture of that!).

Sir William Osler, your belief is again confirmed! It is indeed important what sort of a person has a disease. And Ted was—and is—a very important sort of a person.

Dr. Arthur D. Wolf is an internist on the senior attending staff of Hartford Hospital in Hartford, Conn., as well as the consulting medical director of Jefferson House (the geriatric division of Hartford Hospital) in Newington, Conn. He has also been in private practice in internal medicine in Hartford since 1959. He received his B.A. degree from Yale University and his M.D. from Case Western Reserve University.

Stroke!

*Alan S. Greenglass, M.D.,
Ted's present physician*

Stroke!—it's an abrupt and harsh word that represents what is often an abrupt and harsh condition, one that, though fairly well understood, can be prevented only occasionally, is amenable to medical treatment only rarely, and makes survival or recovery more a matter of fate and hard work than of anything medical science can offer.

What it is

Known technically as a cerebrovascular accident, stroke encompasses many variations of various causes. In general, however, it refers to the damage caused to the brain by the sudden cessation of blood flow.

The brain, like all other living tissue, is in constant need of raw materials, energy, and waste removal. Raw materials include amino acids and fatty substances necessary for the synthesis of brain tissue and of the chemicals that transmit information within the brain. Energy for the brain's activities is provided by oxygen and glucose, without which the brain would starve. And carbon dioxide, urea, and other waste products must be carried away or they will poison the brain.

The brain is a highly active organ, requiring a great deal of these nutrients and producing a great deal of waste products. It therefore needs a rich blood supply, for it is the blood that, through arteries, carries the nutrients into the brain and, through veins, carries the waste away.

The brain is supplied by three major sets of arteries: the right carotid system, the left carotid system, and the vertebral-basilar system. The carotids, which we can easily feel pound when we check for a pulse, travel up each side of the neck from the major arteries leaving the heart. In the neck, each carotid artery divides into an external and an internal artery. The externals travel up *outside* the skull to supply the eyes and scalp; the internals go up *inside* the skull to form the blood supply of the major portion of the brain, the cerebrum—the source of understanding, memory, speech, sensation, and muscle movement.

The vertebral-basilar system is composed of two vertebral arteries, joining to form the basilar artery, which travels up the back of the neck to the cerebellum and brain stem area. This is where coordination and the nerves supplying the head (ears, eyes, mouth) are centered.

All the blood supply of the body is formed in a lattice and web system. Each successive step in the lattice is narrower and able to carry less blood. Blood from several different arteries may supply a particular piece of tissue in the web.

A stroke occurs when the blood supply to a particular area of the brain is interrupted. The type of functional loss depends on which area of the brain is deprived of blood supply. The size of the stroke depends on both the size of the artery that is blocked (the larger the artery, the more brain is involved) and the ability of adjacent arteries to make up a portion of the blood flow lost.

Why it occurs

There are three major causes of stroke. The most common is cerebral thrombosis (the thrombotic stroke). In this condition, the artery supplying the brain slowly narrows over time until the blood flow becomes inadequate to supply the needs of the brain. This is a similar process to that causing heart attack. The process probably begins many years earlier in life. Usually the walls of our arteries are extremely smooth. But due to a number of possible causes, not all of which are under- (although we know that the shear stresses of high blood blood pressure and the corrosive effects of nicotine are the two most commonly identified), an area of an artery is damaged and roughened. This allows the cholesterol normally in our blood to stick to the rough spot, forming a plaque (the higher the blood cholesterol, the faster this occurs), to which clotting factors and calcium also adhere.

The second most common cause of stroke is embolus (the embolic stroke), a clot of blood, cholesterol, and protein that breaks off from either the wall of the heart or the wall of a carotid artery and travels through the lattice until it becomes lodged in a smaller artery. The formation of an embolus in a carotid artery is similar to the process causing a thrombosis, except that instead of blocking the causative artery, the clot breaks off and travels further downstream. An embolus can form in the heart if the heart is enlarged, beats irregularly, or has been damaged by a heart attack, although the heart is not a common source of stroke-causing embolus.

The least frequent cause of stroke is bleeding through the wall of an artery in the brain. In this case, there is a weakened spot in the wall, which may actually bubble out (an aneurysm). The weakened area is either congenital or caused by a wearing thin over time by high blood pressure.

Different effects of stroke

Now that we know what causes stroke, we need to understand why its effects may vary from person to person. Why does one person have left-sided weakness, another have right-sided weakness and loss of speech, and a third has no weakness but a loss of coordination? The reason is that different parts of the brain control different functions.

As mentioned earlier, the back portions of the brain, the cerebellum and brain stem, are responsible for coordination as well as for control of the functioning of the face and head. A stroke affecting this part of the brain can damage one or many of these functions.

The cerebrum is set up in a reverse fashion from what we might expect—the right side (lobe) controls the left side of the body below the neck, while the left lobe controls the right side of the body. Functions such as speech and understanding are centered in the dominant lobe, which in 95 percent of people is the left one.

Thus, the particular neurologic deficit depends on the particular area of the brain that has been damaged by the loss of blood flow.

Stroke prevention

Most strokes will occur without warning, but that does not mean that prevention is impossible. It should now be clear that although some factors that cause strokes are probably beyond our individual control, the most important causes—smoking, high blood pressure, and cholesterol—*are* controllable. Individuals who either

Stroke!

avoid these factors or act to remove them if they already exist can prevent a stroke, or at least reduce the risk of one.

There is another group of people who may also be able to prevent stroke: those who either have had a stroke warning (a transient ischemic attack, known as TIA) or who have narrowing in one or both carotid arteries. The TIA is a short episode—lasting from minutes to a day—of weakness or numbness in one side of the body, of speech loss, or of blindness in one eye. It is caused by an artery being momentarily blocked and then opening up on its own. (TIAs usually occur in parts of the brain supplied by the carotid systems.)

Narrowing of the carotid arteries can often be detected by a health care professional by physical examination. If the suspicion is there, a series of tests can be done to try to confirm it. If a TIA is suspected of arising from a carotid artery, or if the carotid artery is found to be narrowed prior to the advent of symptoms, either medical or surgical therapy may help prevent stroke. It has been shown that one aspirin per day, which decreases the stickiness of certain blood cells (platelets), can decrease the risk of subsequent stroke in people who have had TIAs. Unknown is the value of this treatment in those who have carotid narrowing but have not had a TIA.

Surgical cleaning out (endarterectomy) of an internal carotid artery can return blood flow almost to normal. The benefit of doing this in all cases, however, has not been proven because of the risks, including stroke, of the operation itself. And often the blockage in the artery is too far into the skull to be reached surgically.

Warnings of stroke in the vertebral-basilar system are not very common, and physical examination cannot provide evidence of narrowing in this system. But even if this were not the case, the use of aspirin has not been shown to prevent strokes in the back of the brain, and these arteries are not reachable by surgery.

Stoke treatment

Unfortunately, once a stroke has begun, medical science has very little to offer except supportive care. Many strokes are "completed" suddenly: by the time the victim knows what has happened, the affected brain tissue is damaged beyond repair. Some strokes are "stuttering": the symptoms seem to come and go, or gradually progress, over several hours or days. In these circumstances we may use anticoagulants (blood thinners), though their efficacy has not been universally proven. Sometimes we are led to suspect that brain tissue around the main area of stroke damage is swollen, in which case drugs such as dexamethasone (a steroid) or mannitol (a powerful diuretic) may reduce the swelling, thereby reducing further brain damage, but cannot reverse the damage already done.

With some strokes, blood will accumulate inside the skull. This is commonly the case when the artery has broken, such as in the third type of stroke discussed above. As in the case of swelling around an area of stroke, this blood accumulation can serve to compress and damage otherwise healthy brain tissue. Sometimes the bleeding will not stop on its own. In both these dire circumstances, surgery may be indicated. It is something to avoid if possible, but it may be life saving if a hematoma (blood clot) can be removed or a bleeding artery cauterized.

Our "treatments" of stroke are few and are not always likely to help. We cannot change what has already been damaged. We can, however, sometimes prevent further damage.

Rehabilitation

Unfortunately, many stroke victims (about 150,000 per year in the United States) will not survive the initial brain damage. An additional number will be left unconscious or so paralyzed that rehabilitation will not be possible. Another group of people will show full, or nearly full, recovery on their own.

The largest group is those who, maintaining sufficient mental faculties and physical coordination and strength, can be trained to use their bodies and minds again. Speech therapy may help them swallow and talk again. Occupational therapy may help them use their fingers and hands. Physical therapy may help them walk or get around with a wheelchair, crutches, or cane.

Rehabilitation may be a long and arduous task. Many people won't respond to it: either the damage to the brain and body is too great to permit retraining and recoordination, or the damage to the psyche and soul is too great to permit the amount of effort needed.

Ted Paullin

At seventy-two, Ted Paullin was an active man, physically and intellectually: traveler around the country and world, university professor, lecturer, and author. After smoking for many years (even after he developed lung problems—bronchiectasis), in 1970 he finally heeded his doctor's advice to give it up. Other than his lung problems, though, he was in good health.

His stroke came without warning. A branch of the basilar artery, at the back of the brain, began to bleed, and a clot formed in the cerebellum. Tissues controlling coordination were damaged, and the buildup of pressure from the bleeding and swelling brain caused a disruption of the parts of the brain controlling consciousness and breathing.

Through the use of medications and the efforts of the neurosurgeon, the pressure in the brain was reduced. Since the cerebrum had not been permanently damaged (again, its blood supply is from the carotid arteries), the intellect—the ability to form thoughts—was preserved, as was the strength of the limbs. But the challenge to his recovery was the damaged cerebellum. It prevented him from being able to move his mouth and tongue in a coordinated fashion: he could not form words, he could not swallow. Nor did he have the ability to balance and propel his body.

Thus, during his rehabilitation, Ted had to learn to do some things that people do naturally, such as standing up without falling over. He had to relearn other functions, such as talking. Some things had to be learned to be done differently from before. Instead of automatically swallowing, he had to voluntarily make the muscles at the back of the throat work. He needed to use visual and sensory stimuli to control the positions of his body—a task made harder by damage done to his left eye during the stroke and by a previous cataract on the right eye.

Each step involved hard work, perseverance, and courage both on his part and on his wife Ellen's part. Stubbornness helped, too. After two months in the hospital, Ted was well enough to go to a nursing home. His tracheotomy and gastrostomy tubes were still in; it would be another month before he could breathe and eat without them. Most of the work lay ahead. He became discouraged, but he and Ellen picked each other up.

Stroke!

Sometimes they pushed further or faster than the therapists thought they should. Several months in the nursing home had given them confidence, albeit in a protected environment. They were determined for Ted to ride his exercise bike to build up strength, weight, and stamina. The therapists were afraid that his lack of balance would cause him to fall, but he rode it. They wanted to walk, to read, to socialize, to travel. They wanted to go to Tanglewood and to professional meetings; they wanted to go camping.

And all these advances meant new needs to be met. They needed the hardware, such as special wheelchairs. They learned whom to talk to and what to say—maybe to push a little bit—until they got what they needed. Ted needed to learn individual coordination and mobility, and they had to learn to work as a team. Ellen needed to be a partner in an awkward dance—in and out of wheelchairs, in and out of the car or plane, into buildings, bathrooms, even tents!

There were many setbacks. Without constant attention and work the gains were quickly lost. Speech and swallowing would deteriorate unless Ted paid attention to them. He needed to think them through, step by step. Aspiration occurred several times; eventually, antibiotics were used regularly to control lung infections.

There were many dead ends, perhaps because they were being overly hopeful or perhaps because they were grasping at straws, always looking for something better. A new stroke specialist came to town—could he help? A meeting was both discouraging and encouraging. No, there's nothing more that science can do, but yes, you've done wonders through hard work. Trying different therapists—maybe one who could help them more than the last—brought a burst of enthusiasm on everyone's part (Ted, Ellen, therapist) but the same need for work. At times, disappointment led to depression. Is this all we can expect? Yes, always new obstacles, unplanned setbacks—a respiratory illness, choking on a piece of food, not being able to talk for a week. Won't it ever be easier? No, never easier. You can't stop or you go backwards, vegetate, atrophy, die. Might Ted have another stroke? Possibly. Could we prevent it? Would he recover again? Probably not.

But it's now been five-and-a-half years—five-and-a-half years for a life that might have ended on a roadside; that might have ended if not for the skills of neurosurgery; that might have ended if not for the artificial feeding solutions, antibiotics, expert nursing care. Five-and-a-half years that would have been empty, lonely, closed, if not for a refusal by Ted and Ellen to accept limitations, to believe with Browning that "a man's reach should exceed his grasp, or what's a heaven for?"

Dr. Alan S. Greenglass has been an internist at the Kaiser Permanente Health Plan in East Hartford since 1979 and is currently its chief of internal medicine. Born in 1949 in New York City, he graduated from Columbia University and from Brown University Medical School.

Appendix

I. Bibliography

Changing Health Care for the Aging Society: Planning for the Social Health Maintenance Organization. Lexington, Mass.: Lexington Books, D.C. Heath and Co., 1985.

Dorros, Sidney. *Parkinson's: A Patient's View.* Cabin John, Md.: Seven Locks Press, 1981.

Farrell, Barry. *Pat and Roald.* New York: Dell Publishing Co., 1969.

Johnson, Eric. *Older and Wiser: Wit, Wisdom, and Spirited Advice from the Older Generation.* New York: Walker and Co., 1986.

Judd, Richard L. "Demographics of the Elderly." *Emergency Medical Services Management Adviser* (an Aspen Publication) 1, 11 (February 1986).

Judd, Richard L., Carmen Germaine Warner, and Mark A. Shaffer. *Geriatric Emergencies.* Rockville, Md.: Aspen Publishers, Inc., 1986.

Reed, Janet. *Wheelchair Workout.* Potomac, Md.: JSR Enterprises, 1986.

II. Suggested Readings
A. On Stroke/Cerebrovascular Disease

Brandstater, Murray E. *Stroke Rehabilitation.* 2d ed. Baltimore, Md.: Williams & Wilkins, 1986.

Bray, Grady, and Gary S. Clark. *A Stroke Family Guide and Resource*. Springfield, Ill.: Charles C. Thomas, 1984.

Broida, Helen. *Coping with Stroke*. San Diego, Calif.: College Hill Press, 1979.

Carr, Janet H., and Roberta B. Shepherd. *Early Care of the Stroke Patient: A Positive Approach*. Rockville, Md.: Aspen Publishers, 1979.

Downey, John A. *Stroke: A Guide for Patient and Family*. New York: Raven Press, n.d.

Freese, Arthur S. *Stroke: The New Hope and the New Help*. New York: Random House, 1980.

Griffith, Valerie Eaton. *A Stroke in the Family: A Manual of Home Therapy*. New York: Delacorte Press, 1970.

Hess, Lucille J., and Robert E. Bahr. *What Every Family Should Know About Strokes*. Englewood Cliffs, N.J.: Appleton-Century-Crofts, 1981.

Hewer, Richard L., and Derek T. Wade. *Stroke: A Practical Guide Towards Recovery*. Englewood Cliffs, N.J.: Prentice-Hall, 1986.

Johnstone, Margaret. *Home Care for the Stroke Patient*. New York: Churchill Livingstone Inc., 1980.

Kaplan, Paul E., and Leonard J. Cerulla. *Stroke Rehabilitation*. Stoneham, Mass.: Butterworth Publishers, 1986.

Longenecker, Clarence E. *How to Recover from a Stroke and Make a Successful Comeback*. Port Washington, N.Y.: Ashley Books, 1977.

Appendix

Rose, Clifford, and Rudy Capideo. *Stroke: The Facts.* New York: Oxford University Press, 1981.

Sarno, John E., and Martha Taylor Sarno. *Stroke: A Guide for Patients and Their Families.* New York: McGraw-Hill, 1979.

Smith, Genevieve W. *Care of the Patient with a Stroke: Handbook for the Patient's Family and the Nurse.* New York: Springer Publishing Co., 1977.

B. On Zone Therapy

Bertherat, Therese, and Carol Bernstein. *The Body Has Its Reasons.* New York: Pantheon Books, 1977.

Corvo, Joseph. *The Best Is Yet to Come.* Croyden, Surrey, England: Bedford Books, 1984.

C. Personal Narratives

Armstrong, April Oursler. *Cry Babel: The Nightmare of Aphasia and a Courageous Woman's Struggle to Rebuild Her Life.* Garden City, N.Y.: Doubleday & Co., 1979.

Colman, Hila. *Hanging On.* New York: Atheneum Publishers, 1977.

Dahlberg, Charles Clay, and Joseph Jaffe. *Stroke: A Doctor's Personal Story of His Recovery.* New York: W.W. Norton & Co., 1977.

DeMille, Agnes. *Reprieve: A Memoir.* Garden City, N.Y.: Doubleday & Co., 1981.

Krupnick, Sam. *The Ordeal and the Rainbow: The Story of a Man's Conquest of Stroke.* St. Louis, Mo.: Ishiyaku EuroAmerica Inc., 1986.

Lavin, John H. *Stroke, from Crisis to Victory: A Family Guide.* New York: Franklin Watts, Inc. 1985.

Prazich, Michael N. *Stroke Patient's Own Story.* Danville, Ill.: Interstate Printers & Publishers, Inc., 1985.

Starr, Fern. *Ordeal: One Family's Experience with Stroke.* New York: Vantage, 1984.

Wint, Guy. *The Third Killer: Meditations on a Stroke.* Abelard-Schuman, 1967.

Wulf, Helen H. *Aphasia: My World Alone.* Detroit, Mich.: Wayne State University Press, 1986.

D. Publications

"The Caregiver's Yellow Pages." In *Modern Maturity* (August/September 1987): 32.

Gaining Ground. A newsletter for stroke patients and their families produced four times a year by the American Heart Association, 7320 Greenville Avenue, Dallas, Texas 75231.

The Stroke Connection. Published nine times a year by the Courage Stroke Network, Courage Center, 3915 Golden Valley Road, Golden Valley, Minn. 55422.

Volunteer Stroke Rehabilitation Program, Inc., Newsletter. 96 Westwood Road, New Haven, Conn. 06515.

III. Additional Information

A. Day Care

Helpful books about adult day care are available from the National Institute of Adult Daycare (NIAD), c/o the National Council on the Aging, 600 Maryland Ave.,

Appendix

West Wing 100, Washington, D.C 20024; telephone (202) 479-1200.

B. Travel Information

Publications

Christianson, Mickey A. *Directory of Recreation Resources for the Handicapped.* Write to 1106 Gonsalves Place, Cerritos, Calif. 90701.

Hecker, Helen. *Travel for the Disabled.* Portland, Ore.: Twin Peaks Press.

The Itinerary: Travel Magazine for the Handicapped. Box 1084, Bayonne, N.J. 07002.

Services

Directions Unlimited, 344 Main St., Mt. Kisco, N.Y. 10549.

Elderhostel, 80 Boylston St., Boston, Mass. 02116.

Evergreen Travel Service, 44th Avenue West, Lynwood, Wash. 98036.

Flying Wheels Travel, 143 West Bridge, Box 382, Owatonna, Minn. 55060.

Guided Tour, 555 Ashbourne Rd., Elkins Park, Pa. 19117.

Moss Rehabilitation Hospital, 12th St. and Tabor Rd., Philadelphia, Pa. 19141.

Society for the Advancement of Travel for the Handicapped, 26 Court St., Brooklyn, N.Y. 11242.

Index

A

Abbott, Robert D., 11n.
Acapulco, 100
Adult Day Care Center, 52, 80-90
AE (George William Russell), 16
Agard, Walter, 16
Alexander Meiklejohn Experimental College Foundation, 12, 14, 48, 49
American Friends Service Committee, 16
American Tragedy, An, 121
Amherst, Mass., 17
Anasazi, 48
Ancef, 143
aneurysm, 157-58
Anthology of World Poetry, 43
anticoagulants, 160
Aruba, 100
Australia, 102, 107, 113, 118, 119, 121

B

Beaulieu, Bernadette, 66, 67, 70-75
Beaulieu, Henry, 66, 67, 70-75, 109
Betty Larus Adult Day Care Center, 80
Blake, William, 55

Bombeck, Erma, 40
Boston Red Sox, 106, 107
Brandeis University, 92
Breadloaf conference center, 101
British Volunteer Stroke Scheme, 76
bronchiectasis, 109, 134, 161
Brooklyn, N.Y., 93n.
Browning, Robert, 164

C

cardiac standstill, 135
caregivers, care of, 94-99
Cartagena, 100
catheter, urinary, 150
Central Connecticut State University, 17
cerebellum, 136-37, 158, 162
cerebral thrombosis, 157
cerebrum, 158
Connecticut Community Care, Inc., 94
Cousins, Norman, 10, 30
CT scan, 137, 142

D

Dana, Richard Henry, 52
"Darius Green and His Flying Machine," 116
Deadeye Dick, 53

Decadron, 136
Denver Broncos, 111
Denver, Colo., 14
"Deserted Village, The," 116
dexamethasone, 160
Dickinson, Emily, 18
　poems by, 3, 14, 20, 31, 37, 44, 56, 100, 108, 117, 122, 123, 127, 129
Disneyworld, 48
Doll's House, A, 98
Dreiser, Theodore, 121
dysrhythmia, 135

E
Easter Seal Rehabilitation Center, 39
echocardiogram, 145
edema, 135
embolus, 157
emphysema, 109
endarterectomy, 159
endocarditis, 144-45
Epcot Center, 48
Erb, Martha Jean 100, 101
Experimental College, 12, 14

F
"First Snowfall, The," 43
Fish, Carl Russell, 15
Fitzgerald, F. Scott, 115
Flagstaff, Ariz., 48
Follett, Ken, 52
Fonda, Jane, 96
Fowler, "M. E.", 120
Foxboro, Mass., 55
Friends Journal, The, 46
French Book-of-the-Month Club, 40

G
gastrostomy, 145, 146
Gaus, John, 15
Goldsmith, Oliver, 116
Green Bay, Wis., 15, 48, 120, 122
Green Bay Packers, 4, 55
Greenglass, Alan, 109, 110, 111, 112, 116
　biographical note, 164

H
Haines, Joan, 67, 69
Halley's comet, 100
Hamilton, Walton, 16
Hartford, Conn., 39, 80
Hartford (Conn.) College for Women, 19
Hartford (Conn.) Hospital, 6-7, 26, 110, 133
Hartford *Courant,* 54, 56, 57, 61, 111, 121
Hartford Stage Company, 98
Heller School (Brandeis University), 92
hematoma, 160
hemorrhage, cerebellar, 137, 139
Hippocrates, 151
Homer, Winslow, 78
Horwitch, Norma, 76, 77, 78, 79
Hutchins, Robert, 96

J
Jefferson House, 30, 31, 34
Johnson, Hugh, 61-65, 96
Johnson, Tottie, 61-65
Joyce, Nancy, 76, 78, 79

Index

K
Kahn, James, 52
Kaiser Permanente, 24-25, 39, 41
Kansas State University, 124
Kansas, University of, 16, 18
King, Martin Luther, 41

L
Laakso, Peg, 76, 79
Larson, June, 69
Lawrence, Kans., 16, 18
Long Beach, Calif., 93n.
Lowell, James Russell, 43
Lowell Observatory, 49
Lurtsema, Robert J., 121

M
MacNeil-Lehrer Report, 114
Madison, Wis., 48, 103, 104
Manhattan, Kans., 18, 124
mannitol, 160
Massachusetts Agricultural College, 18
Media, Pa., 16
Medicaid, 91
Medicare, 25, 30, 35, 38, 39, 91
Meiklejohn, Alexander, 51-2
Middlebury College, 101
Mills, C. Wright, 52
Milton, John, 43
Milwaukee, Wis., 122
Minneapolis, Minn., 93n.
Moby Dick, 115
Murrow, Edward R., 119
Murrow: Life and Times, 114

N
Nafcillin, 143
National Heart, Lung and Blood Institute, 11n.
National Organization for Women, 45
Neal, Patricia, 76-77, 79
Newington, Conn., 24, 30
New Yorker, The, 54, 115
Northeast, 56, 57, 64
Northern Arizona University, 48

O
O'Connor, Josephine, 70
O'Hare Airport, 49
O'Neill, "Tip," 107
On Borrowed Time, 27
"On His Blindness," 43
On Wings of Eagles, 52
Osler, Sir William, 136, 154
Our Town, 30, 60

P
Pacifist Research Bureau, 16
Park College, 16
Parkville, Mo., 16
Passage to India, 96
Pat and Roald, 76
Paullin, Ellen Payne, biography of, 17-19
Paullin, Grace Boyden, 122, 124
Paullin, Marcia, 2, 7, 9, 10, 27, 33, 54, 86, 114, 120, 126
Paullin, Theodore (Ted)
  at adult day care center, 80-90
  biography of, 14-17
  cataract surgery, 40
  diagnosed, 9, 137, 162
  in intensive care, 20-30, 141

in skilled nursing facility, 30-36
rehabilitation of, 162-64
stricken, 6-9
suffers setback, 108-12
surgery on brain, 139
Pet Sematary, 110
pons, 139
Portable Dorothy Parker, The, 114
Portland, Ore., 93n.
Powell, John Walker, 14n
Power Elite, The, 52

Q
Quaker International Seminars, 17
Quakers, 16, 120, 122, 126

R
Rapoza, Gail, 70
Rehabilitation, 161
Reserve Officers' Training Corps (ROTC), 15, 18
River Glen Adult Day Care, 87-89
Roland, Ruth, 83, 94
Russell, Bertrand, 16
Russell, George William (AE), 16

S
School for Scandal, 96
Seriatia marcescens, 143
Smithsonian Institution, 121
Smoking, as cause of stroke, 11
Social/Health Maintenance Organization (S/HMO), 93
Social Security, 25

Star Wars: Return of the Jedi, 52
Steegmuller, Francis, 16
Stroke
 causes, 157-58
 defined, 155
 effects, 158
 prevention, 158-60
 treatment, 160-61
Stroke Club(s), 34, 66
Swarthmore, Pa., 16

T
Talking Books for the Blind, 52, 121
Tanglewood, 46, 120, 163
Thomas, Norman, 18
TIA (transient ischemic attack), 159
Townsend, Lucy, 94
tracheotomy, 142
Trowbridge, John, 116
Twain, Mark, 100
Two Years Before the Mast, 52
Tuchman, Barbara, 40
Turner, Frederick Jackson, 103

U
University of Kansas, 16, 18
University of Wisconsin, 12, 13, 14, 16, 47, 103, 104

V
Vermont, 101, 102
Visiting Nurse and Home Care Association, 111
Volunteer Stroke Rehabilitation Program (VSRP), 75-77

Index

van Doren, Mark, 43
Vonnegut, Kurt, 53

W

Washington, D.C., 126
West High School, 78, 120
Wethersfield, Conn., 66
Wilder, Thornton, 30
Will
  Bryn, 2, 3, 4, 32, 54, 55, 120
  Colleen, 2, 3, 4, 5, 6, 7
  Karen, 3, 4, 5, 7, 8, 10, 20, 22, 27, 33, 34, 65, 101, 106, 110, 114, 126
  Kayden, 2, 3, 4, 31, 32, 54, 55, 120
  Philip, 2, 3, 6, 7, 10, 101

Wisconsin, University of, 12, 13, 14, 16, 47, 103, 104
Wolf, Arthur, 6, 7, 24
  biographical note 154
Wright, Frank Lloyd, 16

Y

Yale Art Gallery, 78
Yale University, 75
Yeager, Jeana, 124
YMCA, 122
Yourcenar, Marguerite, 127
YWCA, 18

Z

zone therapy, 96

About the Author

ELLEN PAYNE PAULLIN was born in Amherst, Mass. and grew up in Manhattan, Kans., where her father was on the faculty of Kansas State University. After graduating from KSU in 1936, she served as executive secretary of the YWCA at the University of Kansas, Lawrence. While there, she met and married Ted, the new instructor in the history department. They spent the World War II years in Media, Pa., among Friends (Quakers) and moved to Newington, Conn., in 1947. While her two daughters were young, Ellen wrote *This Little Boy Went to Kindergarten, Karen Is Three, No More Tonsils!* and, later, *Bonjour Philippine.* She has written a biography of Anne Hutchinson (unpublished), edited *Etta's Journal for the year 1874,* and written for local newspapers and Friends publications. After seventeen years in public relations at Hartford College for Women, she is now retired and writes about the age group she knows best, three score and ten plus.

9